THE BABY MAKERS

THE BABY MAKERS

Diana Frank and
Marta Vogel

Carroll & Graf Publishers, Inc.
New York

Copyright © 1988 by Diana Frank and Marta Vogel

All rights reserved

First Carroll & Graf edition 1988

Carroll & Graf Publishers, Inc.
260 Fifth Avenue
New York, NY 10001

Library of Congress Cataloging-in-Publication Data

Frank, Diana, 1942–
    The baby makers / Diana Frank and Marta Vogel.—1st Carroll
& Graf ed.
    p.   cm.
    ISBN 0-88184-374-1
    1. Human reproduction—Technological innovations. I. Vogel,
Marta. II. Title.
QP251.F683 1987
618.1'78—dc19   87-22903
                                                              CIP

Manufactured in the United States of America

Contents

Preface

MAKING BABIES NONTRADITIONALLY HAS BECOME A WAY OF LIFE for many Americans who want children but can't create them the old-fashioned way. The desire of these primarily older and middle-class individuals to have children is intense, and that intensity shows no sign of diminishing. Indeed, given the present social climate—vast numbers of continually working women, later marriages, and postponed childbearing—and increased reproductive hazards in the American workplace and society, the requests that science and society do something to "give us a child," particularly a blood-related one, are sure to continue loud and vocal.

As we see it, both the desire and the response to that desire are products of several important social forces simultaneously at work—widespread contraception, feminism, increasingly sophisticated biotechnology, and the changing nature of the nuclear family.

It all began with control of human procreation—birth control—and the evolution of the philosophy that all children should be wanted children. Americans today not only have all the technical, medical, and legal means to *avoid* giving birth to a child that is not welcome, they increasingly have the means to produce a wanted child.

"We are building a world of one hundred percent wanted children," says Larry Suscy, business manager of Fertility and Genetics Research, a company that franchises new reproductive technologies. "Every step towards that end seems like a good thing."

Creating children, in what is a radical departure from the historical norm, is bound to create vicious controversy, especially when, as in surrogate parenting, proponents ask society to approve it

1

formally. Who, even among the majority who have babies easily, could be indifferent to Baby M?

Faye Wattleton, president of Planned Parenthood, says in a *Washington Post* article, "Nothing is certain except death, taxes, and controversy over reproductive rights."[1] Those "rights," which in the decades since widespread contraception have referred primarily to the ability to *not* have children, are now increasingly applied to the ability to go to any means to have them.

"There's going to be an upheaval of social context around what human reproduction is," says Dr. Gary Hodgen, director of research at the Jones Clinic in Norfolk, Virginia. "It's been going on for about twenty-five years; it started especially when the oral contraceptive became available. . . . Infertility treatment is not new. But *in vitro* fertilization . . . and all of the related reproductive technologies . . . are an order of magnitude different. [These have] increased tremendously the capacity of individuals to go to *extraordinary* means to serve their ends."

But it is by no means technology alone with which we must wrestle. Donor insemination, for example, has little to do with technology (other than the ability to store frozen sperm, a discovery made in the 1949s). It has much more to do with our cultural definitions of mother and father and with the rights of children to know their biological origins. The same is true of surrogate motherhood. Alternative reproductive technologies force us as a society to deal with fundamental questions. But even when we reduce matters to a dispassionate manipulation of sperm and egg, few thinking people find the issues easy to handle.

Ultimately, reproductive technologies and the uncomfortable questions they force us to face—how far we should go, who will have access to them, what is for sale and what is not, who is the "real parent," how to balance individual and social rights—will not go away. The discussions will not be easy or dispassionate but the issues must continue to be addressed. The how and why and who of having babies involves political, spiritual, cultural, and emotional questions of overwhelming importance.

A Word About Language and Names

The language of reproduction has always carried special potency, whether uttered as insult or with the secretive kind of giggle that talking about what people do behind closed doors evokes. You can't say "sex" to someone without bringing up a flood of connotations—good, bad, but never indifferent.

Science and reproduction also have a mutual history of powerful meanings. It was, perhaps, the label of "test-tube baby", applied to Louise Brown, the first child conceived in a glass dish, that, more than the procedure itself, aroused deeply held fears that science had come to control what previously had been the private business between a man and a woman. *Donor insemination* (DI) is an example of how grappling with the language involves grappling with our emotions and beliefs about a process we've never felt at home with.

But it's the simple words *parent* and *mother* and *father* more than the scientific labels that in particular will continue to be redefined controversially in light of new ways of reproducing.

The old definitions of *mother,* where biology, genetics, and nurturing were, in most cases, conveniently rolled into one, lack the fine-tuning needed for the high-tech mother whose job description may include only one or none of those functions. The so-called "ovum transfer," "adoptive pregnancy," or "prenatal adoption," for example, where eggs and genes are scrambled between women, presents a particularly complex linguistic challenge. Is the mother the one who carries the child? Is she the one who donates her egg? Or is she the one who breast-feeds the child (as some *adoptive* mothers do now)?

"You ask me biologically who is the mother?" says Norfolk's Dr. Zev Rosenwaks. "Technically, biologically, the genetic mother is the egg donor. There is no ambiguity there—the genetic material is the egg donor's. On the other hand, the woman who carries it, nurtures it, is really the mother—biological mother, not genetic mother. She carries it, she nurtures it, takes it to term, delivers. Certainly you can't convince the women who carried the children that they're not the mothers."

But definitions get trickier when another kind of "motherhood" comes into play, where nurturing and shaping the baby are not included. Surrogate kingpin Noel Keane coined and appropriately massaged the term *surrogate mother* to make a point. Combined with the help of the highly visible "Phil Donahue Show," the term *surrogate* helped win "surrogate" mothers official recognition. The less-than-real, stand-in nature of the term *surrogate* conveniently flipped attention away from the traditional nurturing, shaping functions of the woman who carried the baby (the role the doctors have unflappably used as the criterion for motherhood in "ovum transfer") to the nothing-proceeding-it "mother" who brings up the child.

As the public tries to formulate what it really thinks about having a child by some other method than the "traditional," it is important to recognize that words are no small part of the process. The public relations campaign to make people comfortable with what they might otherwise feel squeamish about clearly works. While the catheters, petri dishes, and microcameras of science allow the bodily vessels to be probed and plucked, it is the all-important tool of *language* that persuades the head and the heart to proceed.

Some detachment may be necessary, but we should not so gently and dispassionately use language that, in order to ease our pain, distorts reality. Despite the advances of technology, the truth is that a man and a woman—at least some part of each of their being and spirit—are still needed to create a child.

As an illustration of the potency of the subject, many of the people we interviewed have requested that we give them a fictitious name, to protect their own identity or the identity of their child. These are, in all cases, couples or singles who are recipients or donors of reproductive services. In all cases, doctors, researchers, and other professionals have been correctly identified.

The terms you will come across most frequently are: DI, IVF, and surrogacy. We've taken some liberties with the first term, DI, to describe insemination by donor. In the literature it was, until recently, and by some people still is, frequently described as AID—artificial insemination by donor. Because of the confusion with the term AIDS (acquired immune deficiency syndrome), we've chosen to use DI. In the interest of further reducing confusion, we've taken the liberty of substituting DI for AID in quotes and in places where others have referred to AID.

In vitro fertilization, or IVF, is the process of uniting a sperm and an egg in a petri dish outside the human body. *Surrogate motherhood* is the process of artificially inseminating a woman who is not the husband's wife with his sperm. When *in vitro* fertilization is used to mix the woman's egg and her husband's sperm and the fertilized egg is then implanted into another woman, we use the term *in vitro surrogate* to indicate that the woman is carrying a child to which she has not genetically contributed.

In the process of researching this book, we interviewed more than one hundred scientific researchers, physicians, administrators, couples, singles, etc. In no way do we suggest that this is a scientific survey. These people were selected because they best represented and expressed the feelings and sentiments that arise in connection with what is a highly personal topic. Though we would like to have spoken with more men, it remains true that the subject is largely a female area of interest.

This book is not, as most others published have been, a consumer's guide to the infertility market. Nor is it an exhaustive survey of the causes and treatments of infertility. *The Baby Makers* deals with the personal, medical, and social response to issues of childlessness. The majority of people with reproductive problems are helped before the newest reproductive alternatives become necessary. Those who have children by means of DI, IVF, or surrogacy have usually tried more conventional therapies first. DI is generally the last option for couples where the man is infertile; IVF has primarily been used in cases where the woman has obstructions in the reproductive system, but recently IVF has also proved useful for men with low sperm counts. Surrogacy is normally the solution for women who have gone through years of medical treatments—and sometimes attempted adoption—and still do not have a baby.

While this book is grounded in our research into the new technology, we make no pretense of presenting the most up-to-date discussion of actual treatments for infertility. Our reason for writing is simply to uncover legitimate questions required for an informed discussion of the subject in general.

Chapter 1 explores the social background of why couples go to such intense trouble to have children, and what children mean to them.

Chapter 2 explores the intricacies and social ramifications of donor insemination, a "low-tech" procedure that is the basis for other procedures.

Chapter 3 explores *in vitro* fertilization and the trials and tribulations of infertile couples considering IVF.

Chapter 4 explores the history and the intricate scientific world around IVF.

Chapter 5 looks at the blossoming industry of high-tech babies.

Chapter 6 explores the last resort of infertile women—surrogate motherhood and its history and ramifications, from the couples' viewpoint.

Chapter 7 looks at surrogacy from the viewpoint of the surrogate, the woman who receives money for giving up a baby.

Chapter 8 explores the growing business of surrogacy and the agencies that have made it possible.

Chapter 9 looks at the moral/ethical questions inherent in surrogacy and the new reproductive technologies. These are questions often *not* explored by the infertile but explored by politicians, the churches, and the ethicists.

1

Why Children?

IN HER SIXTH WEEK OF PREGNANCY IN 1979, SHIRLEY WILLIAMS, a thirty-one-year-old secretary, woke up at six in the morning and crumbled to the floor, bleeding profusely.

Williams had a tubal pregnancy—probably caused by some kind of birth defect—on the part of the fallopian tube that enters the uterus. The fetus had literally exploded her womb. By the time her sister got her to the hospital, Williams' veins had collapsed and she almost died.

By December 1980, after several emergency surgeries and two more attempts to clean out and reconstruct her fallopian tubes, Williams was hoping to start another pregnancy, thinking that her tubes were now in working order.

She asked her doctor, "When can I try to have children?" He answered, "There's no way it's really going to work. The surgery was not successful, and you're just going to have to live with it." There was no way egg and sperm were ever going to meet in her reproductive tract.

Like many infertile couples, Williams and her husband were desperate to have children. Years earlier, they would have had to bear their grief quietly and perhaps attempt adoption, but by 1980

7

the options for someone like Williams were expanding, and she wanted to explore them.

Williams was aware that a so-called test tube baby girl had been born in England in 1978 to Lesley Brown, whose tubes, like Williams', were blocked. She also knew that a few surrogate babies had been delivered and relinquished to infertile American couples. In 1981, Williams heard that the first American test tube baby was born at Norfolk with the help of a procedure involving the removal of a ripe egg that was then fertilized in a petri dish (*in vitro*) and implanted into the womb of the would-be mother.

Still, for Williams, finances and the not-quite-perfected technology were serious considerations.

"At the time, *in vitro* fertilization was far out of the picture," says Williams, "because insurance wasn't taking care of it. It was a money factor. We just didn't have that kind of money—six to eight thousands dollars."

Instead, Williams entertained the idea of hiring a surrogate mother, a concept that was just catching on.

She learned about Noel Keane's program on a television show called about the surrogate program, and was "absolutely appalled by the prices and what you didn't get." She was worried that the surrogate mothers were not sufficiently aware of what they were doing. "I thought that no matter how psychologically adjusted one could be, anyone who walks through the door and says, 'Hi, I'm Mary; I want to give somebody a baby,' needed to be talked to," says Williams.

A few years passed and Williams was still desperate for a baby. In 1985, by which time *in vitro* fertilization (IVF) had become better established, Williams' home state, Maryland, passed a law requiring insurance to cover IVF.

In spite of having reached the point where she "couldn't stand to be cut open one more time," Shirley Williams nevertheless decided that if doctors came up with a way to get her pregnant, she would tell them, "Just get your knife out and cut another hole."

When her physician told her, "You're a perfect candidate for IVF. You have great ovaries, there's nothing wrong with your uterus," Williams decided to go for it.

"I just knew in my heart, that if I kept at it, I had all the parts except the tube, and the doctors had the answers to all the rest," says Williams.

Seven months and four embryo implantations later, Williams was pregnant.

Still, it took her a while to comprehend her luck.

"You just don't believe it; you don't buy into it for a long time

. . . I didn't buy the first article of baby clothing until I was seven months pregnant because I thought terrible things would happen." Williams remembers thinking, "Tomorrow I'll wake up and all this will have been a dream."

Terrible things did not happen during the pregnancy, but the delivery by cesarean section was full of unpleasant surprises. "Normally a cesarean takes thirty to forty-five minutes, but because of all the adhesions from my previous surgery, my bladder and a host of other organs were literally pasted to my uterus, so they had to cut all those adhesions and we were pushing two hours," Williams recalls. "There were three doctors, and when they plucked the little turkey out, he was blue, not breathing."

The baby was rushed to another hospital specializing in neonatology. He survived without suffering any damage, and Williams was put back together again. Both had been in grave danger.

"For ten years, all I wanted was one child," says Williams, who never thought she would "be greedy about this." Now she confesses, "The baby wasn't back from the hospital for two days when I was saying to my doctor, 'I want to go do it again.' "

The Williamses are saving up for another child. This time, if the doctors refuse to risk Shirley's life again, it will be a baby born of a surrogate mother.

Not everybody is as lucky as Shirley Williams. Some people with fertility problems struggle for years and eventually have to give up.

Psychologists who have studied infertile people assure us that grief over "the loss" of a child not even conceived is almost identical to the grief over the death of a close family member.

Cathy Cheleen, writing in Washington, D.C.'s *Resolve Newsletter* (November 1986), wrote this obituary: "Erin, the little girl with the musical talent from her father's side of the family, her mother's love of books and reading, and curly auburn hair from both sides of her family, died in the doctor's office. Her death was not particularly sudden or unexpected. The results of numerous tests were not good, and yet her family was not prepared for her death. . . . Her 'death' came when they, and their doctors, came to the conclusion that they were an infertile couple."

The longing for a child conjures up complete human beings with specific features and special talents. These wished-for children are like little actors waiting in the wings for the doctor's cue calling them into the light to play their role in the lives of their parents. When the doctor fails to call them forth, they vanish into the darkness; their bones disintegrate along with their parents' hopes. But there is no coffin, no flowers, no letters of sympathy.

"It is strange," Mark Jacobsen, who had a run-in with infertility, wrote in *Esquire*[1], "that when you're trying to create life, death is so often on your mind." He recalled an evening with fellow sufferers who had given up and were going to adopt.

"I didn't want to be around people who'd tried and admitted their failure. I said I had to get something out of the car. On the way out I passed a window with very colorful furniture inside. I looked in. It was a kid's room. It was all set up; it looked like it had been there for some time. It was like peering into a mausoleum."

A diagnosis of infertility is devastating to people who want children. First there is shock and disbelief, often followed by denials. "Please, doctor, don't say we are infertile. It's just taking us a long time to get pregnant. Please don't say infertile," was how Cindy and Tim Connors, a Kensington, Maryland, couple with a four-year history of childlessness, reacted to their doctor's diagnosis.

Infertility can shatter people's notion of reality and leave them disoriented. One woman told Barbara Eck Menning, the founder of Resolve (a support group for infertile people), "When my father died suddenly in the night, twenty years ago, I remember that for months afterward his death seemed unreal. I'd wake up every morning thinking: 'Nothing had really happened. I dreamed the whole thing. I'll go to my parents' room and find them both there.' I experienced the same confusion with my infertility. It felt like a bad dream. Nothing had changed in my everyday life: No one had died, no one was sick, everyone looked the same. *Yet everything had changed.*"[2]

Bargaining with God and fate for a child rekindles hope for a brief flash. Said one barren woman, "It seemed to me that there was no amount of pain I wouldn't undergo gladly in exchange for a body that could make a baby. Maybe that's what fertility rites and ritual sacrifice are all about. I'm an educated woman of the twentieth century, but emotionally I guess I'm not much different from my cave-dwelling ancestors."[3]

When deals with fate do not work out, deep depression and despair are likely to set in. One sufferer who could not cope with her feelings of sorrow said, "For a long time, I have tried to push myself to keep functioning. I would never commit suicide, but often I have wished that I would get hit by a truck so I wouldn't have to endure it anymore."[4]

Finally, for those who get that far, there is acceptance of reality. The long struggle with infertility makes some people much more understanding of other people's suffering, but for a minority it ruins their lives. Says Susan Mikesell, a psychologist in Washington, D.C., who counsels infertile couples, "Having to come to terms with the fact that they can't do anything about it is really very painful. A lot of people walk away much more cognizant of how difficult it is to have what you want in the world; they come to have much more of a sensitivity for people struggling with something. Some are very cynical, like 'I was deprived of this. It wasn't fair. I didn't do anything.' Some people have a really bitter response that they never get over totally.''

In the past, adoption was the only "cure" for childlessness, but modern medicine now keeps barren people in suspended animation as it offers them hope in the form of a huge array of treatments, including fertility pills, surgery, artificial insemination, and *in vitro* fertilization. Infertile couples "are frequently driven," says Dr. Gary Hodgen, director of research at the *in vitro* clinic in Norfolk. "They are obsessed with the issue of having a child. They turn to the physician and they say, 'Do what you can for me,' and then when it doesn't work, they say, 'Turn it up higher and do more. Give me high tech; we've got to have a kid.' "

The hoped-for children of the infertile are the objects of obsession—planned for, plotted for, prayed for, and paid for. A child conceived by the most novel methods, *in vitro* fertilization or surrogacy, usually strains both the parents' emotional endurance and their pocketbook. Even so, the hardest part comes after the birth.

A Boston woman who chose not to have children was quoted in *Newsweek* as saying of her friends, "They all wanted to experience maternity, [but] some of them hadn't thought of what it would be like afterwards. Now they all dearly love their children, but many of them have said that if they knew beforehand what was involved, they might have decided not to have any.''[5]

A child born in the 1980s will cost its parents at least $150,000 to raise. To be able to afford children, often both mother and father have to work full-time, which necessitates day-care. Most working families spend 10 percent of their income on child care. Although a child is often considered the glue that holds a marriage together, quite the opposite is often true. A newborn is likely to cause a strain on the marriage; statistics indicate that the rate of divorce is highest after the birth of the first child, and, according to UCLA researcher Bonnie Burman, couples who remain childless by choice rate higher on a marital-happiness scale than parents.[6] Besides that, the child may not prove such good company. Twenty-one percent of people surveyed by the British magazine *Options* preferred their pets to their children.

If kids are a drain on a couple's energy, bank account, and emotional resources, why, then, do people want them?

That question is relatively new, for as one mother, a mother of three children, says, "In my day, nobody asked themselves whether it was worth it or not. In my day, you just had them, for God's sake."[7] Still, today, when we have almost full control of our fertility, people rarely ask themselves the questions before the children arrive. Even infertile couples who have struggled with the how for years give little thought to the why, probably because answers are so deeply imbedded in biological, social, and psychological realities that it is difficult to come up with an answer.

"For me, it was something I always wanted since before I was married . . . since I was eighteen years old," said one infertile woman. "I think it is sort of instinct—that may not be the right word."

Instinct may not be the right word, but it does point to a very real drive that goes beyond reason—our bodies are programmed to ensure the survival of the species.

"Survival," says Germaine Greer, "is one of these occult motivations, and when our hormones gush in response to external stimuli which become more effective because the hormones are agush, the ancient, inveterate will of the species is being done, for the nadir of unfitness to survive is 'inability or unwillingness to breed.' "[8]

The will of the species manifests itself in an individual desire for children of one's own. "I believe one of the main purposes of life is passing on your DNA, and that is certainly the only purpose of life among the lower species," says Steve, a very successful businessman whose wife is infertile. "I didn't feel comfortable in not taking the ultimate steps I could to fulfill my biological destiny. . . . I have an I.Q. of 150 or above; I have been very successful in life. Part of that can be passed on." Steve is now trying to get a surrogate mother pregnant.

Susan Mikesell feels it is the continuation of one's genes through the generations that spurs people to act. "Many a couple has come in here—not necessarily infertile couples, just couples I work with—talking about the decision about having children when they are dealing with parents who are ill. How they really hadn't thought about having kids in their life and then it is like 'I really don't know if I could *not* have a child.' It is dealing with the loss of that generation and moving on forward having those connections on either end. . . ."

Writer Richard Cohen understands this urge. "My wife and I have one son of our own, and one of our pleasures is to talk about his ancestry—the Koens of Poland, the Fitzgeralds of Ireland. It is even a greater pleasure to see some of my wife and some of me in our son—and also, sometimes, to see my father's smile on my son's face. Anyone who does not understand that is disconnected from humanity."[9]

In the past this emotional response to a biological imperative translated into the idea of dynasties, but even today pride in the family and its accumulated possessions becomes a reason for having offspring, preferably boys.

Elena Ringger told *Newsweek* that when her only son, forty years old, announced that he intended to remain childless, she was stunned. She wanted a grandson to inherit the large family home and the forty-four photo albums she had assembled over thirty-five years. "I remember asking in a pique: What the hell am I making these albums for? What is going to happen to the family name? . . . I feel cheated."[10] she said. The older generation's wish for grandchildren is its way of dealing with its own mortality, psychologists say. Grandchildren make this world a little bit easier to leave. As long as we are remembered, we are not entirely absent from the world of the living.

In the propagation of the human species, families have traditionally held a central role. People got married and were ordered by the church "to be fruitful and multiply." "Kids—that's what I thought marriage was all about," says one infertile man. A couple without children do not a family make, it seems, especially in modern society, where the definition of family has shrunk. "I think now that people are more isolated from their extended families, there is a sense that the tiny nuclear family needs its own child to justify its existence," says psychologist Dr. David Glass, who counsels infertile couples in Arlington, Virginia. His view is echoed by Mikesell: "The more upwardly mobile individual couple is removed from the extended family, [it is] just the two of them. With the nuclear family being their base, there is a lot more pressure to have a child. . . . In the extended family in the past, you had your sister's children; her kids might be as much yours in some ways because you were involved with their growing up."

It has always been a man's role to provide sperm and a woman's to supply an egg and a womb in the creation of a family and a new generation. "A person who is not able to fulfill that basic human function of supreme importance may feel inadequate as a human being, as a man or a woman," says Glass.

Although anthropologist Margaret Mead maintained that male sexuality seemed to have no goal beyond "immediate discharge," many men are eager to have children, not necessarily because they enjoy the pleasures of child-rearing but because the basic ability to have a baby confirms their masculinity. If a man cannot have children, his self-image may suffer. Said one infertile man, "I feel emasculated. I can make love to my wife ten times a week, but she and I both know I'm only shooting blanks. I'm sterile, and that makes me feel impotent."[11]

Bringing a child into the world is one of the developmental milestones on the road through life, a sort of rite of passage between childhood and adulthood. A man is just one of the boys until he fathers a baby, and a woman may not consider herself fully grown-up unless she has given birth.

Sex and its consequences, children, have always been the touchstone of a woman's life. They can both ruin her and add to her worth.

The Talmud says, "A daughter is a vain treasure to her father. From anxiety about her he does not sleep at night; during her early years lest she be seduced, in her adolescence lest she go astray, in her marriageable years lest she does not find a husband, when she is married lest she be childless, when she is old lest she practice witchcraft."

Whether a woman had children or not, the question of progeny was always fundamental.

Until contraception came along in the beginning of the twentieth century, female premarital sex was not only a father's worry, it was dangerous business for women. Should pregnancy result from illicit intercourse, there were, until less than two decades ago, only three real options: a shotgun marriage, a back-alley abortion, or going away to have the child and then putting it up for adoption. The rare woman who chose to keep a child born out of wedlock was severely compromised socially.

A woman who had a child before marriage was a creature to be pitied, but the same was true of a married woman who failed to produce babies. A childless married woman was a worthless wife. Women were little more than reproduction machines for men who knew the value of private property. A previously "owned" woman could be had at a reduced price, whereas a girl with an unbroken seal guaranteeing, there had been no tampering with the product, was worth incomparably more. Having acquired a suitable piece of property, having made an investment through marriage, the man expected it to yield reasonable returns, a decent number of children.

The idea of the child as a product was set early on. Notes Germaine Greer, "The value of women has virtually never involved their personhood, but rather has involved their being used as a means to achieve valued economic ends. It is probably no accident that the Church came to support the virtue of chastity inordinately for women. As bearers of children, feudal social organization focused upon the children produced by women rather than on either the marital relationship or the value of women as persons."[12]

The view of women as wives and mothers reached its apotheosis in the Victorian era, when those roles were the only possible foundations for female identity. Since the only form of safe birth control was "moral restraint," which it was up to their husbands to exercise, married women seemed almost perpetually pregnant (if they did not die in childbirth).

Women have made great strides in their own liberation, but the Victorian view of women, although eroded, is not dead. It coexists with the idea of women as participants in "the man's world." Men have little interest in seeing women as competitors in the job and income market, but women, although unwilling to admit it, are probably also afraid to let the traditional role disappear completely. It is a fallback position; if you cannot hack it in the man's world, there may be the option of maintaining self-worth and a means of survival in being a wife and mother. So far there has been little attempt by American society to fuse career and family roles, and women find themselves on a procrustean bed, being pulled in two directions at once. To be a wife and a mother is fine, to be a career woman is fine, but being both is pretty near impossible. Men as husbands generally want children, but men as employers generally do not. Employers have been known to say, "A pretty little thing like you ought to be home having a baby every year," implying that since they do not like to grant maternity leave, the woman ought to stay home and be a wife and a mother.

In a effort to downplay women's "biological destiny," feminists began to devalue motherhood and stress career goals as more worthwhile in life, and many women began to see themselves as members of their profession first and as mothers second. Financially, women became independent of men, but on another level they bought into the man's world, they assumed a man's values and rearranged their priorities according to the rules of his world.

There was a time, a tiny blip in modern Western history, when, given the perceived importance of what used to be a job and now became a "career" to women, liberal attitudes about sex, and the widespread use of contraceptives, some women experimented with the radical idea of remaining childless.

In 1960 only one out of ten married or divorced women between the ages of twenty-five and thirty-four was childless; by 1986 the ratio was one out of four—a total of nearly 3.3 million women. Women, who are often financially penalized for having kids have good reasons for postponing childbearing. Harvard economist David E. Bloom found that the income of woman managers with similar educational backgrounds varied according to whether they had children or not. Women managers with children made about 20 percent less than those who had remained childless. A Stanford University study showed that for all working women, wages decrease with each additional child. Fathers' earnings, on the other hand, are not affected by the number of children they have. Bloom predicts that 30 percent of all woman managers will remain childless.[13]

But while more and more couples decide to remain childless, the idea is threatening to the very core of society. "In many societies," says Greer, "the notion of human accountability to posterity is at the heart of the entire moral system. The group must be advanced by one's participation, in material terms, in spiritual terms, and in terms of growing larger and more powerful, be it the family, the tribe, or the nation. . . . It is not advanced at all by childlessness."[14]

The social pressure on couples to have children is strong. One childless woman said she knows that some people who have made a decision not to have children "lie and say they are still trying when people ask them why they don't have kids. Childless couples often gravitate towards other childless couples; there's no need to be defensive with people who have made the same choice."[15] Writer Gael Greene, writing "A Vote Against Motherhood" in the *Saturday Evening Post*, received letters full of pity: "Seeing your children grow into happy, useful people—graduating from the best colleges on the honor roll—producing grandchildren who put their arms around you and tell you that they love you . . . This will never be your privilege." She also received letters of outrage. Readers called her all manner of names, such as "a spoiled and selfish woman," "a shriveled and stunted personality," even "judging from your horrible photograph . . . a worn-out prostitute."[16]

The childless woman, especially the barren woman, has always been a kind of social outcast, identified by everyone who knows of her affliction and pitied more even than someone with a visible deformity.

The first generation of feminists made great strides in changing social attitudes and encouraged women to pursue careers more eagerly than babies, but now the second generation, which not only grew up with the new idea of a woman's role but takes it for granted, wants it all: career and motherhood. These women seem to have come around again to Margaret Mead's opinion that "full acceptance of responsible life in society is having children."

Early feminists condemned motherhood as bondage and as something only a woman could do and thus demeaning, but now it has become something only a woman can do and thus spectacular. Women can have both career and baby, as attested by the "Woman at Work" clothes for executive women with a briefcase in hand and a baby in progress.

The current drive to have children is, in many ways, a combination of old and new pressures—the ancient pressure on women and men to fulfill their biological destinies, the evolution of the feminist mandate to control one's world as well as one's body, and consumer pressure to have a child as an indication of status.

Many of the people who feel the pressure to produce offspring have sufficiently explored the world of work and are now ready to explore the less well-defined world of children. But a substantial number of women who put off having children, choosing to further their careers instead, bumped into an obstacle they had never anticipated. It was something for which nothing in their pursuit of career had prepared them: infertility.

"There is a confusion, a feeling of being duped," says Mikesell of career woman who have learned that success lies in proper management. These women, says Constance Shapiro, an infertility counselor in Ithaca, New York, "have essentially lived with the belief that if you plan, if you're achievement oriented, think ahead, and try to do things right, having a baby is something that should simply happen when you decide, just as a degree should. All the experiences they had have prepared them to think that if they try hard enough, they will experience success." Therefore, a diagnosis of infertility is "a substantial jolt" and commonly accompanied by feelings of "overwhelming grief."

The misery of the infertile can hardly be exaggerated, but the pain of a childless couple in the West does not compare with the pariah status of the barren in preindustrialized societies. Greer mentions a village in Egypt where ten childless women "were known by everybody . . . Two were living with husbands who had taken a second wife . . . The fact that childless women retained their looks was considered in itself sinister. The villagers said: 'A childless woman is usually like a she-camel who does not conceive, puts on more flesh and gets younger every day'—but not fruitful, she can never 'lengthen her husband's neck' among the menfolk. She is an eyesore to her family.''[17]

Among the Aowin of Ghana, "the sterile man or woman is never fully accepted as a member of society. Barren women are suspected of being witches. Men who have no children are called derisive names and at a funeral of a childless person, the corpse is abused as the mourners instruct the spirit of the dead never to return again.''[18]

At the same time, because there is little a couple in these societies can do about their infertility, their affliction is stoically endured in a way that infertility in America is not.

In more primitive societies infertility is perhaps deemed God's decision and hence intractable. But Americans are not so quick to take God's decision as the last word, especially where medical science is involved.

"We have a knack of turning everything that bothers us into a problem, a problem being something for which there must be a solution,'' says New York psychologist Bernie Zilbergeld. "We have great faith in solutions and have refused to accept the possibility of insoluble problems, the very idea being contradictory to many of us.''[19]

As a consequence, the last few decades have seen many infertile people determined to solve problems of conception by resorting to radical solutions such as artificial insemination, *in vitro* conception, and surrogacy—solutions that the general public may feel uneasy about because they challenge established feelings and ideas about procreation and family.

2

Donor Insemination: Surrogate Fathering

"I THINK THE THING I WAS MOST NERVOUS ABOUT WAS HAVING A baby by . . . some strange man, an anonymous person," says Martha, a thirty-six-year-old private school teacher who had a child through donor insemination about three years ago. "That was a very anxious thing for me."

By the time she was thirty-two, she and her husband, Dave, had been trying for two years to get pregnant. Then they discovered the "big shocker": His sperm count was too low. After discussing the matter, they realized that there was little choice; Martha would be inseminated with another man's sperm.

Somewhat apprehensive but desperate for a child, Martha and Dave visited the sperm bank, where row after row of numbered, heavy steel jugs with lids that read, "Caution—do not lay on side," lined the room. This is where, when what happens in the bedroom fails, the couple or the doctor acting in their behalf—or sometimes a woman acting on her own—comes in search of a suitable replica of the husband (or of a lover or even of an imagined ideal). The liquid nitrogen steams up like the witches' brew in *MacBeth*. The specimens are kept in the cold darkness, just below the surface, at −196 degrees Centigrade. With an "extender solution" added to prevent ice crystals, the sperm are in suspended animation. They can stay that way for perhaps ten years and still "father" a baby. One Danish donor reportedly had sperm stored for twelve years that resulted in a birth.[1]

Martha and Dave's physician picked out a donor who looked like Dave. Martha kept her temperature charts to show when she was ovulating and got hormone shots every time the doctor inseminated her. It took several months and several attempts before she got pregnant.

"[There was] uncertainty, real uncertainty," says Martha. "And the fact that we had to put our faith in a total stranger, this doctor—he's making a selection that we had no control over. I probably slept only half the amount I usually would. My big worry was that I couldn't be too sure about this baby. I remember being about five months pregnant and waking up in the middle of the night and having what I thought was the closest thing to a spiritual bond with the baby, and the words that came into my head were, 'Who are you?' "

There are about thirty sperm banks in the United States, but you won't find any of them listed in the Yellow Pages. The majority of inseminations—75 to 85 percent—involve fresh semen, even though the American Association of Tissue Banks says frozen is safer because it can be quarantined for sixty days and thus guaranteed to be AIDS-free. The Idant Sperm Bank in New York City is believed to be the largest in the world, with over 30,000 specimens. It has sired an estimated 11,000 babies since 1971. The collection and distribution of sperm to women—donor insemination (DI)—has proceeded without interruption for years, but "the procedures of DI have been cloaked in secrecy," says Dr. Armand Karow, president of Xytex Sperm Bank in Georgia.

"The original reason we were located in this area, in the lower level without windows," says Roxanne Feldshuh, codirector of the Indant Sperm Bank in New York, "was because of the fear that we might be a target of some sort." Powerful social and religious forces kept DI from being something that, if it was done at all, people wished to talk about or record.

Although DI with humans is mentioned in the Talmud in the fifth century A.D. and in Spanish documents in the fifteenth century, there is only slight evidence of this practice in early history. DI evolved from its use with farm animals, where its success was more probable, given that while human ejaculate may contain 200 million sperm, a bull produces 10 billion sperm.[2] Economic considerations make it advantageous to use one prize bull's sperm to inseminate many cows. While there was little outcry about toying with the reproduction of cows, applying the same technology to humans was another matter, unless, of course, for the benefit of a soldier husband, in which case the sperm would have to be stored for some time. In 1776 it was discovered that some human sperm survived freezing. In 1866, Montegazza, an Italian scientist, "speculated that in the future . . . frozen semen might be used not only in breeding the finest farm animals, but for saving the sperm of a man going off to war so that his wife might have a legitimate child from him even though he died on the battlefield."[3] It was an interesting theory at the time but held little hope in practicality, as less than 10 percent of the sperm survived.

In 1884, in the most celebrated case of what some might call a kind of sexless rape, Dr. William Pancost at Jefferson Medical College in Philadelphia decided to "assist" the wife of a rich Philadelphian merchant who was having problems getting pregnant. When he examined her and saw that she was perfectly fertile, he chose the best-looking student in his class, asked for a "donation," anesthetized the woman with chloroform, and inseminated her. When the child was born, the doctor told the merchant what had been done, but the mother remained ignorant of the facts.[4]

Using medical students as a sperm source became the norm early on. In 1949, with the discovery that glycerol helped many more than 10 percent of the sperm live, the technology responsible for the development of modern sperm banks took a giant leap forward. The first sperm bank for humans was established in 1954.[5] Freezing was introduced in 1953 and the first American child was born of frozen donor sperm in 1954. In 1960 in the United States, an estimated 5,000 to 7,000 DI children were born, possibly more, as records were not kept accurately, but as late as 1974 the American Medical Association still deemed the procedure "experimental."[6]

Introducing the child-producing liquid of an anonymous man, into a woman he is not married to is "experimental" and "secretive" because it threatens deeply held cultural values. Some whisper of adultery. Some grandparents, when the truth is revealed, withhold inheritance from the non-blood-related child.

In a kind of silent, institutionalized ceremony, mediated by the medical community, a man and a women who will never meet agree to produce a baby who will probably never know its biological father. The traditional vehicles—sexual love and sexual intercourse—have nothing to do with this conception. The man, separated from his contribution except for a three-digit number, does not think the word *father*. Because he is not required actually to have intercourse with the mother, he can detach himself and not think about the fact that he may pass his son or daughter on the street someday. Because of this same detachment, sanctioned by the scientific community, the mother only has to think about his eye color or his hair and hope that it is the same as her husband's.

"I mean, it's not a stranger, it's semen," says Margaret, mother of a DI child. "I don't even conceive that there was sort of a person on the other end before it got to be semen. No that didn't even occur to me."[7]

In adoption, the doctor explained to Hillary, a DI recipient, when she asked if she should tell the child, are were other people involved; there is a relationship. In this situation, there is just a donation—an offering of sperm given the way you make a contribution of money to Goodwill.

DI is distinctly a "low-tech" process, requiring little more than a syringe. Doctors preside in an established kind of ceremony. It's a timed affair on the woman's part. If the body is not as predictable as medical science would like, a sonogram is used to pronounce her follicles ripe and the doctor tricks the body into ovulation with drugs. The frozen straws of sperm are thawed at room temperature. The doctor injects "the donation" near the cervix on what he thinks is the day before ovulation. The cost is typically $60 a straw, with two straws used per insemination. (The do-it-yourself special requires only a turkey baster and a friend.)

Religious Opposition

The Catholic Church has opposed DI because it requires masturbation—an "intrinsically and seriously disordered act" and a "deliberate use of the sexual faculty outside normal conjugal relations [which] lacks the sexual relationship called for by the moral order [which is] self-giving and [aims at] human procreation in the context of true love.' "[8]

In 1951 Pope Pius XII condemned donor insemination on the grounds that it "converts the domestic hearth, the sanctity of the family into nothing more than a biological laboratory." The Catholic Church may have seen even then that, although DI was technologically simple, its practice and acceptance laid the foundation for other babymaking procedures. DI was the first technique developed using a third person to create a child; it officially allowed someone else to be involved, however anonymously. It coaxed procreation out of the bedroom and into the doctor's office, and it made babies only half-related biologically to the parents officially more acceptable. It introduced the idea of selling the procreative services of the body to an unrelated person.

DI set the stage for *in vitro* fertilization by allowing sperm to be separated from its donor and sequestered, at least temporarily, in the laboratory. (While the term *artificial* had long been applied to insemination, it was the birth of Louise Brown that brought that word to the headlines: "An artificially conceived baby: It's an epochal event in medicine's annals and could hasten even bigger— and more disturbing—breakthroughs."[9] But it's questionable which is more artificial—a baby who is produced through the egg and sperm of his own parents, united outside the body but "reintroduced" to the mother, or a baby who is produced by putting the semen of an unknown man into the vagina of the mother.

Donor insemination may also be seen as the flip side of surrogate motherhood. Tania, one DI mother, says that "surrogate mothering has only been happening for about six years and in a way it's more open" than DI, which she refers to as "surrogate fathering."[10] In surrogacy, the woman "donates" her egg (unless she is a "surrogate womb" only) and her body; in artificial insemination the man "donates" his sperm. The man receives $30–$50 for each "acceptable" donation, while the woman generally receives $10,000 for a delivered baby. In surrogacy, the legal mother adopts the child; in DI, in many states, the "social" father is *assumed* to be the legal father and no adoption is necessary.

Dr. Sherman Silber, author of *How to Get Pregnant,* likens DI to adopting sperm—"the only choice in a sense is to adopt the baby at a much earlier stage, i.e., prior to conception."[11] But for many people, while DI is still something that may be necessary, it is not the kind of thing most people want to talk about. Canadian sociologist Rona Achilles cites studies which concluded that while community attitudes toward new reproductive techniques were generally quite positive, DI was viewed as "the most problematic."[12]

For everyone involved in this, the oldest unregulated process of producing a portion of the future's children—the wives, their husbands, the donors, the doctors, and the children—there are intermingled questions, concerns, fears, and hopes. Sometimes these are expressed but more often they remain wrapped in a secrecy that suggests society's profound ambivalence. Most people involved in this large system of unknowns will express a lack of interest in knowing about the other players; the few voices of those who articulate the questions others are too afraid to talk about illustrate the fragile nature of any consensus about DI. How do doctors feel about hand-picking the children of the future? Why do donors donate and how do they feel about it? How do women feel about carrying a stranger's baby? How do their husbands cope with another man's child? How does a child feel upon learning that the man her mother is married to is not his or her biological father? These are questions that the medical community, for the most part, is not interested in exploring. They stir things up and may upset a system whose functions largely depend on people not thinking about it too much.

When Martha asked her doctor about support groups for women who had used DI, he said, "Lady, I think this is something you only want to discuss with your husband."

The Donors

Five thousand healthy men a year, 40 percent of them medical and dental students from nearby universities, enter the doors of the Xytex Corporation sperm bank in Augusta, Georgia. They are predominantly white, young, with few sexual partners and no homosexual experiences. They are, for the most part, under age thirty-five. Sperm from older men, it turns out, entails the same risks as eggs from older women.

"It was always thought that the woman was at a greater risk of Mongoloidism," says Dr. Jerome Sherman, director of the Semen Cryobank at the University of Arkansas and chairman of the American Association of Tissue Banks (AATB) Reproductive Council. "But the man has a greater risk, too [at age thirty-five]."

Since there is so much demand for the right stuff and since so little of it qualifies, often the first question of a donor is, "Do you have a college education?" Educated sperm have the corner on the market. Notes Idant's Feldshuh, "One of the criteria is always intelligence and some documentation of achievement in an academic sense. . . . By far, the most important question, given that this is a healthy person, is intelligence."

The Repository of Germinal Choice, a sperm bank whose donors include Nobel Laureates, is in business to produce "a few more creative, intelligent people who otherwise might not be born," but most sperm buyers will settle for a little graduate work or a college education.

The majority of donor applicants are disqualified because their sperm flunk the freeze-tolerance test. Sperm attrition or sperm death is a problem. If the donor's sperm passes, he gets $50 in Georgia, $30 in New York. Xytex, when it opened in 1976, accepted one in ten to one in fifteen. Now it takes one in forty. "An acceptable donor [one whose sperm can be frozen and thawed and still be considered fertile] is admittedly not a 'normal' individual," says Xytex president Dr. Armand M. Karow. "We aren't accepting the average person walking in off the street."

The regulars donate once a week or once a month, but always there are at least three days between donations. The donors at Idant, as elsewhere, are predictable. Banks can rely on their sperm count and on the motility and quality of their sperm. Quality is so predictable, says Feldshuh, that if a donor hasn't abstained or isn't feeling well, there is no point in making an appointment—he won't be paid because chances are that the quality won't be there.

The average donor fills four to five plastic straws (some fill twelve), which look something like a coffee stirrer and hold half a cubic centimeter (cc.) of semen. The straws are rushed to a small metal cylinder specially designed for slow cooling. In about forty-five minutes, the sperm will be frozen at −130 degrees Fahrenheit.

Bruce, a sperm donor, says he donated to one bank and was accepted but a year later was rejected at another. The sperm's motility was fine, the speed was fine, they said, but the sperm weren't swimming in one direction. His lackadaisical sperm, they maintained, were "not goal oriented."

Karow is not sure why some men's semen can withstand the freezing and thawing process and still have 55 million motile sperm cells, the number he guarantees the doctor. (The lower limit of normality is 20 million sperm cells, of which 60 percent are motile.)

According to Roxanne Feldshuh, of Idant, if there is a large percentage of abnormally shaped cells in the ejaculate or if the semen is very viscous, it does not freeze properly. "And some sperm are just fragile," she says. "There are changes in the membranes of the sperm."

As sperm banks go, Xytex has a slight puritanical streak—the men who donated the first four years received "no visual stimulus," and if they were married, they were required to have their wife sign a statement that she approved.

"We're conservative enough to think what marriage is about—the wife has a right to voice her opinion," says Karow. Lately, Xytex has loosened up, permitting "visual stimulus," and the husband, if he chooses not to tell his wife, can sign a statement to that effect.

Who are these men who take time out from a job to undergo extensive tests, who go to a medical office to "perform," who make a few bucks providing children they will never see?

The recipients know little about the donors, but Martha has given considerable thought to the biological father of her child. Her pregnancy, she says, was "a horrible state of anxiety. When that baby was born, he was tall and he was a low birth weight for his height—seventy-sixth percentile for height, fifteenth percentile for weight."

She believes that her anxiety about the unknown father may have contributed to the baby's low birth weight. Martha thought about the donor frequently and had dreams about him. "Oh, yes. I fantasize about that all the time. I was wondering if he [the doctor] gave us this information to, in a way, steer us away from the actual guy. I knew that he [the donor] had a northern European background—Danish and German. I know he is six foot one; I know that he has perfect pitch and he plays the French horn and that he is probably part of the Mormon clergy and that he is married and has a family of his own." Later she learned that he is the biological father of fifteen or sixteen children.

But while Martha and other mothers of DI children may wonder about the stranger they will never meet, the donor in this secret ceremony is the Rodney Dangerfield of the system—a bit player, necessary for the play to go on, but lacking full status. Though the bodily fluids of these "DNA providers," as Idant calls them, are precious to those who receive them, the anonymity of the system requires that no one delve too closely into the whys and wherefores of their choosing to play in this game.

"If anything, donors are not given enough respect," says Barbara Raboy, director of the Sperm Bank of Northern California. "Most people who work at sperm banks who recruit donors don't take the time to find out about donors as individuals. They just give blood tests and pay them. They don't get into discussions about their feelings."

Sperm banks may not be the place to talk about feelings, but most donors, though they may have given it little initial thought, have, over time, considered their part in the process.

"No one is going to come to us without having thought about it," says Feldshuh, "knowing what the implications are and being humanitarian to some degree, feeling that he is contributing to the genetic pool by helping couples—or however he phrases it for himself."

"Most of them are doing this because they had a friend who couldn't have a baby," says Xytex technician Pat Harrell. "Our donors are really looking to the idea that they're able to help."

Sixty-six percent of the donors at the Sperm Bank of Northern California said the reason they donated was "altruism." Thus, Karow's donor recruitment—he's taken to advertising to women, suggesting that they tell their male friends to contribute—emphasizes the "helping concept." But Achilles dug a little deeper and found most often a combination of reasons—"never just one reason"—including, initially at least, a sexual kick, the money, wanting to help, and wanting to pass their genes on.

For Nelson a donor, who said it was "almost a joke, a kick being paid to do this,"[13] and for whom the idea seemed ludicrous initially, continuous donation over time in the detached environment of the medical office becomes disillusioning. For Robert, a twenty-six-year-old unmarried postal worker, "it was a kind of joke at first. I didn't really need the money . . . but to get paid for masturbating . . . [laughs] . . . plus the fact that it was sort of like a sexual thing, too—that the nurse knew what you did. I know it sounds terrible. The thing is, at the clinic they act so clinical and I try to act as clinically as them, but sometimes when I am alone in that room I start laughing because I can't believe it, thinking of myself like Tom Selleck or somebody."[14]

But Achilles reports that the sexual nature of the donations soon wears off.

"It was all really clinical and like you'd never talk about what exactly was happening," notes Nelson, a graduate student. "Because of the bizarreness of the situation, I just felt supreme alienation. . . . This whole thing had been a sexual thing, until then it was suddenly a medical procedure . . . I'd never see anyone . . . like 'Mission Impossible'—'Go to room thirty-three.' It wasn't like this nice place to masturbate; it wasn't sexual at all . . . it was like this job. The sense of doing it for someone wasn't really there. It was really removed, partly because I was getting paid. It made me feel creepy. It became incredibly alienating."[15]

At AAA-rated sperm banks, there are soundproof walls; at less particular facilities, the accommodations can be barren and the attitude, says one donor, is like "Give us a urine sample."

One donor recalls a room that was dark and dingy, and there was a sign on the wall: "Due to faulty architecture, lab noises come through walls. If you find this distracting, try running the water. If it still is distracting, we can move you to an examination room."

Reports Robert, "To go into a room and to see men's magazines lying on a sofa, it's sort of degrading sometimes. You feel like a little teenager sometimes going in there—like your mother sending you, like you've been a bad boy . . . and you have to go in there by yourself. And, you know, what you do is sort of like an immature act really. I used to [masturbate] for the fun of it. After going through that program, it struck me that there was a purpose for that and to do it just for the enjoyment . . . well, I feel guilty now."[16]

Getting paid for the donation is generally positive. For example, Larry, a thirty-three-year-old salesman who wasn't "looking for financial gain," said, "I think the financial thing may have sweetened the thing."[17]

But for some men, associating money with a precious part of creation may become distasteful after a time.

Nelson stopped donating (at least partly) because the payment made him feel "creepy" and alienated. "If you give blood, you know you're doing it for someone, but this was different; part of it was the money. . . ."[18]

Tom, the divorced father of two children through marriage, said he would donate without pay. "It's like being a blood donor as far as I'm concerned—it's the same thing. But also, I wanted to get my lineage out. It's really not important what the name is, but I think I would like to have my genes carry on." When reminded that he already had two children through marriage, he replied, "Yes, but it gives you greater chances, doesn't it?"[19]

Achilles says the motives are "an impulse to reproduce, which is distinct from the desire to parent." For single men without children, DI may be a way to sow their seed. As Achilles notes, "DI was perceived by them as a way of mitigating their unmarried and childless state." Drew, a thirty-one-year-old policeman who was not paid, said, "I think there is a bit of immortality involved in having offspring, even if you don't have a relationship with the lady . . . even if I don't know about it. At least I'll have children."[20] He also said, "God, I could start my own country."[21]

Robert, the twenty-six-year-old unmarried postal worker mentioned earlier, described the experience in terms of a "power trip," an "ego trip," for which he considered himself a "study." "It was great that people think of me highly enough to want me to be part of their family history. It's mind-boggling to me."[22]

The Women

"The first time I was inseminated I was very scared. My legs were shaking," says Hillary, a twenty-eight-year-old nurse. "It was kind of frightening. That night when I went home, as I was trying to fall asleep, I remember crying because I felt like I had done something wrong. I felt like I had been unfaithful to my husband. He reassured me that I hadn't done anything wrong." Hillary has told no one that her two-and-a-half-year-old Terri is the product of a visit to the sperm bank.

"I have to laugh to myself when people know I'm trying to get pregnant and they say, 'Oh, I guess you're going to run home and have fun tonight,' " says Hillary. "I had heard people mention DI. Someone said, 'That's awful; I could never do that.' I didn't want to tell anyone and have them pass judgment on me, because this was my personal decision. They thought it was immoral."

The doctor wrote down "all kinds of special talents that my husband had, so they could get the best possible man. That made me feel much better about it."

After four months she did not conceive, but on the sixth cycle she got pregnant but miscarried. Six more cycles went by, and then the doctor found she had antibodies against her husband's sperm.

"My doctor hypothesized that if we had sex on the nights I was inseminated, my husband's seminal fluid would kill the sperm," says Hillary. So they abstained from sex two days before and after the inseminations. Finally she conceived and carried the pregnancy.

Hillary received the sperm of donor number 238, but it wasn't until two months before delivery that she called to find out that his hair was brown, his ethnic background was German, his height was six feet, and his blood type was O positive.

"I worried," she said. "I told my husband, 'What if the baby doesn't look like us; what will people say?' He said, 'Nobody knows what the baby is going to look like; I know families where their children don't look anything like them.' "

Women like Hillary and Martha who bear DI children carry special fears, special griefs, and special secrets. Their first problem, in a society that has traditionally "blamed" the woman for the lack of children, may lie in trying to get their husbands to get a sperm count.

"I get some women calling up, and it is really pitiful," says Anne Kranz, who does telephone counseling as a member of the infertility support group Resolve. "Their husbands don't want to have anything to do with it. That is hard for me to hear. Either it's too painful for them or they are just terrible men or they feel too threatened themselves. I personally know one couple where the man refuses to get a sperm count."

"Nothing bothers me more," says Dr. Martin Quigley of the Texas Health Science Center in Houston, "than a wife having gone through a complete evaluation, including biopsies, laparoscopies, hysterosalpingograms, perhaps several trials of clomiphene, only subsequently to find out that her husband has a severely low sperm count."[23]

Once the inadequate sperm count has been acknowledged, the child that will never be born must also be acknowledged.

Martha explored her feelings in sessions with a therapist. "One of the things you have to get over and the reason it's a little complex is, there is a kind of death of the baby you will never have with your husband. Because you don't see that baby ever, you're mourning, and sometimes you don't know why. My therapist helped me to visualize the baby we never had, and to take the baby in your mind to a very peaceful place and dig a hole in the ground and put it there. A good place, a place where it could rest. That was really helpful."

"It has been a bigger thing for the wives, interestingly enough," says therapist Constance Shapiro. "The women don't quite believe the men when they say it is okay to go through this. Their dream when they married him was for the baby to have his curly hair and his blue eyes . . . and they need to grieve a bit that this baby [conceived through donor insemination] comes to them without being exactly what they had fantasized, but usually it is that the wives want to be really sure that the husbands are telling the truth, because they are terrified they will have this baby and their husband will reject it."

The bonding for Hillary came slowly. "I thought he was kind of funny looking, but I didn't say that to anybody. When I had him at home and was nursing him, he seemed like such a stranger to me—I didn't know anything about him and thought, who is this little child? But those feelings passed. It took a week or two. It was very gradual.''

Both Hillary and Martha and their husbands want a second child by DI. They are going through the process again, this time with a little less apprehension.

The Husbands

The husband is the odd man out of donor insemination. He is the reason his wife has to resort to this and can do nothing but stand by and wait for her to bear another man's child. Although he is unlikely to say much about it, in a society where fertility is still very much associated with masculinity, the very process may stir up deep doubts and fears in him.

Achilles spoke to three husbands, two of whom had had vasectomies, and noted a "reticence to speak about their experience—a reticence that may reflect the difficulties their role involves both socially and emotionally."[24] With both adoption and surrogate motherhood it is obvious to the outside world that the woman is not bearing her biological child. Given the relative openness of these conditions, compared to DI, many couples don't bother to hide the fact. But what Achilles calls the "social invisibility of paternity and assumption of paternity within marriage"[25] makes the "surrogate father" situation more likely to be kept secret.

George, a donor, wonders "if the secrecy is purely for the sake of the husband—to protect his frail ego. . . . I would say that if anybody requires psychological counseling of any kind it has to be the husband; I would imagine his pain is great. . . . In a male-dominated society with male-dominated attitudes toward the getting of children, the man is supposed to be, quite frankly, all balls and cock. That's the whole attitude, and if that doesn't follow, he is less than a man—he is the third sex. He is not man enough by society's arbitrarily applied rules to be a father."[26].

The psychological impact of a diagnosis of male infertility can be devastating.

"I would rather tell a man that he has cancer than that he can't reproduce,'' says Dr. Joseph Lanasa, a New Orleans male infertility specialist. "Men can't separate their hormonal function from their reproductive function. The testes have two functions: one, to produce hormones, the other, to produce sperm. When you tell them that they are not going to be able to reproduce, it really affects them. You have to spend a fair amount of time counseling them.''

Tim Connor's inept sperm was a shock to him. ''I could do anything I wanted and did anything I wanted, and suddenly I couldn't have the thing I wanted the most—children.''

When Tim and his wife Cindy contemplated donor insemination, he did not take to the idea. ''My geneology was very important to me—having a little Tim was important to me—and I didn't want to consider it an option for a long time,'' says Tim.

For Hillary's husband, Roger, the verdict of infertility was not a total surprise. Roger was born with an exposed bladder, a problem that was surgically corrected when he was only fourteen months old.

''They had to reconstruct literally everything,'' he says. ''It was always amazing to the doctors who treated me that I could lead a normal life. I was a miracle patient and I was thankful for that.''

But there were residual problems. When Roger ejaculated, the semen did not come out of the penis but went back into the bladder—a so-called retrograde ejaculation. After an orgasm, his urine was clouded and full of semen. Normally when a man has an orgasm the sphincter muscle clamps shut, preventing urine access to the penis and letting the ejaculate pass instead. Sometimes the entrance to the bladder fails to close, in which case there is a normal orgasm but nothing comes out. Certain medications, like antihypertensives, can weaken the nerves controlling the muscle, and surgery on the bladder or prostate can also cause the condition. In Roger's case, it was part of his general bladder problems. At age sixteen, the retrograde ejaculation is was taken care of by surgery.

Although the operation was successful, he was still plagued with infections of the epididymis, where the sperm is stored. ''A lot of swelling and a lot of pain,'' he says. The infections were regularly treated with antibiotics, but there was permanent damage. Roger's semen analysis showed that the ejaculate had no sperm, or ''aspermia,'' a condition present in only about 4 percent of the overall male population. The doctors suspected that infections had obstructed the narrow coil in the epididymis, trapping the sperm.

In some cases the obstruction can be removed or the sperm can be detoured, according to Lanasa, with relatively new techniques not commonly available six years ago when Roger's problem was diagnosed. Also, the doctors suggested that Roger's blockage, "could well be in more than one given area," making surgery a doubtful remedy. Although the doctors offered him the chance of surgery, Roger decided to accept his infertility.

For those men to whom the reason for having a child is "blood," the lack of such a tie to a child may be devastating, especially since it is something his wife has while he does not. This leads couples like Rev. Deborah Kappe, a Presbyterian minister in Chicago, and her husband to choose adoption over DI because both want to have exactly the same relationship with the child.

DI may strain the relationships between the child and the father. "For the husband," says Dr. Joseph Blizzard, himself a "social father" to a donor offspring, "DI might have a deeper psychological effect than if he and his wife decided to adopt a child."[27]

After two years of marriage, Blizzard discovered that he had aspermia, failure of the sperm to form or to be emitted. DI was suggested and commenced within a week of diagnosis. Blizzard's wife became pregnant and gave birth, but, notes Blizzard, "we have a child who rectifies the moments of despair but, oh dear, does she have a load on her little shoulders."

Blizzard went into profound depression. "I have been unable to sustain even the most facile dialogue with friends. My career is currently in jeopardy. Recreational activities have stopped. I seem to have aged thirty years in six months. The pregnancy has been a continuous statement of my infertility. Next time I'd try something else."[28]

Then there is the unexpressed feeling of competition with another man, alluded to by Martha's husband.

Larry, a donor, wonders "whether going through the pregnancy makes up for the fact that some other man's sperm is in their wife—how do they cope with that? I think . . . a couple would have to do an awful lot of soul searching; it would have to be a pretty open-minded husband."[29] Frank calls it a "patent admission of failure as a man, for the couple to resort to this kind of *institutionalized cuckoldry*. I think their decision marks courage and unselfishness."[30]

Nevertheless, thousands of fathers every year get past the lack of biological connection and love the child in the same way that thousands of adoptive parents do. In fact, Hillary's husband bonded with the baby even before she did.

"When the baby was born, my husband bonded with him intensely, immediately," says Hillary. "He said he was so adorable and he felt proud and he just felt love for him immediately. I asked him, 'Do you feel any reservations about DI?' and he said 'No.' "

The Lag in Male Infertility Research

The traditional attitude that the inability to produce a child is a female problem has left research on male infertility light years behind the study of female reproduction. Whereas women are treated by specialists in gynecology and obstetrics as well as reproductive endocrinology, men have to bring their problems to a urologist for whom infertility used to be a minor side show.

"Ten to fifteen years ago," says Dr. Lanasa, "all physicians did was to tell them that it will take time and to take some thyroid extract and you will get your wife pregnant." (The thyroid gland regulates the metabolism, and a superactive or a subactive thyroid can interfere with sperm production, but the condition is rarely allowed to get bad enough to cause infertility.)

The impetus to study male reproduction came from economic interest in animals. Dr. John MacLeod, one of the few physicians to specialize in the metabolism and cytology—the structure, function, and life history—of sperm when it was not a popular area of medicine, received much of the money for his early research from Cornelius Vanderbilt Whitney, not because Mr. Whitney was infertile, but because one of his race horses was. A stallion in the Whitney stables, Boojum, "was turning out to be something of a flop at stud," said Dr. MacLeod, who promised to take a look at the problem. Dr. Macleod's research had indicated that vitamin B complex helped infertile men, so he supplemented Boojum's feed with it. Boojum got three of four mares in foal and Mr. Whitney liberally supported Dr. MacLeod's human research for the next fourteen years.[27] But there were not enough Whitneys to go around.

"When I started in graduate school in sixty-nine, people were just starting to put some serious research and some serious money into male infertility," says Dr. Jane Chihal, a Dallas, Texas, fertility specialist. "Now there is a lot of good work going on, and I think it has a lot to do with attitudinal changes."

"I now see men sooner, and I'm seeing less reluctance on the part of the man," says Dr. Lanasa. "Occasionally, I see a man come in here because his wife closed her legs, saying, 'You're not going to bed with me until you go and see a doctor.' That gets their attention. I see some that come under duress, but that's a rare occurrence; I see more willing to be here. They are willing to take an active part.''

The "blame" for infertility is now agreed to be equally shared between the sexes. According to Dr. Bellina, 35 percent of the time the problems can be traced to the woman, 35 percent to the man. In about 20 percent of infertility cases the problem lies with both of them, and in the remaining 10 percent the cause is never found.[28] Other estimates place male infertility at 40 percent and men as a contributing factor in an additional 20 percent of cases of inability to conceive.

Testing and Treating Male Infertility

Exactly the same brain hormones that regulate the female reproductive system, follicle stimulating hormone (FSH) and luteinizing hormone (LH), control the production of sperm. In men the target of the hormonal signals is the testicles. In women the hormones are switched on and off in monthly pattern, but in men they are released simultaneously in a steady stream. Only FSH is directly involved in sperm production.

The male hormone testosterone helps develop the reproductive organs in the fetus and causes the organs to enlarge at puberty. Testosterone, also responsible for the characteristic male musculature, is necessary for the sex drive, but it seems to play only a small role in actual sperm production. Apparently a little testosterone goes a long way, and too much "closes down the factory," as Dr. Bellina puts it. A man with all of society's signs of virility— bulging muscles and a never dormant sex drive—may well, for all his outward show of masculinity, be sterile and "shooting blanks." The highest sperm count ever recorded at Dr. Bellina's Omega Institute belonged to a man who stood about five feet five inches, weighed 135 pounds, and had no hair on his chest.

Men are normally fertile around the clock and seem to have an inexhaustible supply of the "right stuff," even though it takes approximately three months to make the tadpole-like sperm.

The fundamental sperm generators, and there are several million of them, are called the spermatogonia, or mother cells. They are located in the testes, which are housed in the pouchlike scrotum. Although it seems a vulnerable shelter for such important ingredients of life, there is a reason for the precarious location. Sperm production requires a temperature three or four degrees lower than the normal body's 98.7 degrees. By hanging away from the groin, the testes avoid overheating. It is for this reason that men with fertility problems are told to forego tight underpants or jeans, which may press the testicles against the body and "overcook" the sperm.

The mother cells make duplicates of themselves, spermatocytes, and send them on their way, dropping them into the center of the tubules, the hundreds of wrinkled threads coiled together in the testicles. The spermatocytes divide, making two types of cells, those needed to make baby girls and those needed for boys. They are now called spermatids and they eventually grow into full-fledged sperm.

The mature sperm are stored in the epididymis, hollow coils on top and on the sides of the testicles, where they can survive for about a month. Some of them move into the vas deferens, a tube (which is cut during a vasectomy) that leads from each testicle to the penis.

Sperm make up only about 2 percent of the ejaculate. The rest is seminal fluid, which comes from two seminal vesicles and the prostate gland. The viscous quality of the 2–4 milliliters of ejaculate helps it stick to the vaginal canal and the entrance to the cervix. At the same time it impedes the sperm's ability to swim. To overcome this, a chemical from the prostate gland causes the sticky substances to liquefy about twenty minutes after ejaculation, so the sperm can get on its way.

Tests to determine a man's fertility rarely involve greater hardship than the slight embarrassment of masturbating into a cup while looking at pictures in *Playboy*. And yet that may be asking too much in some cases. Some men become extremely upset, and Dr. Joseph H. Bellina has seen more than one man faint when asked for a specimen.

Analysis of the semen, including color, viscosity, and sperm count, can tell the physician a great deal about a man's problems.

"We are very careful about our semen analysis," says Dr. Jane Chihal, in Dallas, Texas. "Most places find them frankly boring. They don't specialize in the area, and they miss a lot of problems we pick up."

Under a high-powered microscope, drop by drop, technicians grade the swimming ability of the sperm on a scale from 0 to 4—0 implying no motion at all, and 4 the ability to swim in a straight line with good power. They take another drop and, with a solution of formaldahyde and salt, fix the sperm in place so that they can be counted. Finally they take a look at the shape, the morphology, of the sperm. Even in a normal sample, about 40 percent of the sperm is deformed—having two tails, a blunted head, not fully developed, etc.—and therefore unable to impregnate a woman.

"The rule of the 60s," defining the lower limit of normal sperm, states that men with under 60 percent motility, under 60 percent normal forms, and less than 60 million sperm per ejaculate will have a hard time impregnating a woman. Men with lower counts have fathered children, but the chances of conception are greatly reduced.

"Often they just give you a sperm count," says Dr. Lanasa, "and numbers are the least important factor in a semen sample. The single most important factor is the sperm's motility, the ability of the sperm to swim, and it has to be observed over a period of time. You look at it initially, at one hour, and at two hours. Most labs only look at it initially. We find several men have good motility initially, and then after two hours, it is extremely poor."

If the sperm do not survive for long, there may be something wrong with the seminal plasma or the prostate, or there may be antibodies in the semen.

"If there are sperm antibodies present, the tip-off is that you see vibratory or shaking motion during the semen analysis," explains Dr. Lanasa. The sperm may also clump, agglutinate, in the woman's cervical mucus in response to antibodies, which interferes with their motion. Antibodies, a common problem in men who have had vasectomies reversed, can be eliminated by separating the seminal fluid, the source of the antibodies, from the sperm. In some cases the problem of sperm antibodies be treated with steroids, but this does not seem to help men with reversed vasectomies very much.

One problem with sperm research, notes Chihal, is that "it takes a long time to make a sperm. If you start fertility therapy in March, it is summer before you know if it had an effect or not. It is a very difficult process because of the lag time between treatment and being able to evaluate the result."

Speculation about rising male infertility points to stress of the rising population density, (which has been shown to increase infertility in animal populations), environmental pollution, and drugs combating ulcers and colitis.

Low sperm count may also be caused by a varicose vein, a varicocele, on the scrotum. Coughing will make the veins in the scrotum swell, and the physician may be able to see or feel a vein that swells too much. Doctors have found that 30–40 percent of all infertile men have a varicocele, but they are not sure how that may reduce fertility. One theory is that the warm blood that pools in the veins causes the sperm factory in the testicles to overheat and kill the sperm. The cure is to surgically tie off the bulging veins.

When Matt, age thirty-five, and Betty Peterson, age thirty-two, both professional writers, decided to have a baby, they suspected they might have a problem in spite of repeated reassurances from doctors.

Due to a childhood disease, one of Matt's testicles had been removed, but the other one was, according to the physicians, able to do the job. When, after many months of trying, Betty did not get pregnant, Matt had a semen analysis and found that "the sperm counts were far lower than necessary for a reasonable chance of getting a pregnancy."

"I felt betrayed by the doctors who had handled me as a youth and who had assured me so many times that, even though I had only one testicle, there would not be a problem." Matt had to face reality. "Oh, it was a terrible blow—like I was letting down the woman I love. I felt very guilty that several years into the marriage suddenly my wife found herself with someone who wasn't going to fulfill part of the marriage vow, part of the marriage obligation, part of the joy of marriage."

As is often the case, Matt's low sperm count affected their sex life.

"For me," says Matt, "it was a constant reminder of failure, and there were times when Betty had to remind me that the time was right, let's do it. It was frustrating because there was a part of me that didn't want to do it. It was mechanical, it was like going through the motions—what's the point?" But the doctor gave him some hope when a varicole was discovered and treated.

Some men have demonstrated a dramatic improvement in their sperm quality after a varicocelectomy. A study done between 1963 and 1975 by the New York urologists Richard Amelar and Lawrence Dubin included 986 men who underwent varicocelectomy. Four hundred sixteen of them had sperm counts above 10 million per milliliter of semen before surgery. Eighty-five percent of those men improved after the operation, and 70 percent of them were able to impregnate their partners. For the rest, who had counts under 10 million per milliliter, only 35 percent showed better semen quality and a scant 27 percent obtained a pregnancy.[33]

The varicocelectomy helped Matt Peterson's sperm count some and gave him the sense that he was participating.

"I was glad to have the surgery because I was glad to have some of the pain. It was the one pain I could have; otherwise it was always Betty [who later went through *in vitro*]. I was hesitant to push it to the next step. It was unfair. It was kind of up to her because it was really her going through it. Many tearful times I told her, I wish I could bear all this.''

After the operation Matt was also put on Clomid—$250 worth. His sperm count went up substantially.

If administered properly, according to Dr. Lanasa, hormones can be useful in men "who have good counts, but poor motility. That's where hormones may be effective, particularly if they have low testosterone and low LH levels. Those men benefit from human chorionic gonadotropin [a hormone that resembles LH], and if they also have low FSH, they also benefit from Clomid use.''

Matt had some viable sperm but not enough, so he began giving semen samples to a sperm bank, which froze several portions of his ejaculate in order to save up for enough volume to inseminate Betty. However, freezing usually kills some of the sperm and lessens the motility of the survivors to some degree, and it also reduces longevity to half that of fresh sperm.

Betty did one round of artificial insemination by her husband's sperm and did not get pregnant. They abandoned further attempts when it became apparent that Matt's semen did not freeze well.

They considered artificial insemination by donor but decided against it, Betty being more against it than Matt.

The Sperm Distributors

Martha and Dave's doctor is a "pretty controversial character.'' He "chooses men who are married and have their own family,'' says Martha. "First of all, because that's proof that they produce healthy children. This doctor has a very Nazi-like mentality, and those are not my words. . . . He's done a lot of research in genetics and I think an ego may be involved there. He made some racist remarks while we were there. He has seven criteria for screening, seven tests for hereditary diseases. Height is one of his criteria. He says tall people are always chosen for leadership. There can be no cases of mental illness in the family. He also uses IQ for a criterion.''

If ever there were to be a case made that man is playing God, it might be made with the physicians who quietly pick bits and pieces of the future generation.

The doctor who told Martha, "Lady, I think this is something you only want to discuss with your husband,'' reflects the silence with which the selection and procedure is carried out. Despite her repeated attempts to interview them, sociologist Rona Achilles found that physicians were largely unwilling to cooperate.[31] Not many in the medical community want to talk about what they do.

The matchmaker/doctor peruses his catalog for a proper match. Unlike in *some* surrogate mother situations, where the couple may meet with the woman, couples who choose DI put their trust in the person with the white coat.

At Idant, upon receipt of the doctor's request form, the sperm bank staff searches through the computer, for example, for all Italian men with blue eyes who are six foot or more. The staff takes pictures of the couple to match with a donor. The couple, however, has the ultimate authority to declare a match acceptable.

The form the couple signs before the selection says that they "understand the doctor cannot be held responsible for any physical or mental characteristics of any child so produced. At the moment of conception the husband must automatically accept the child as his own."

While it may be a bit frightening to leave the selection of your child by donor to one who relishes the control, there is also, as Martha notes, a bit of comfort in knowing that you have purebred progeny.

"In a way, while I don't like people to have the kind of mentality he did," says Martha about her physician, "in a way, that was consoling—that he wanted these kids to be so superior just from a health standpoint. It was good to know all these things. . . . He's chosen donors who have what he says are neutral features so that they don't cancel out any of the mother to a great degree."

DI is as much a numbers game as other reproductive technologies, especially when age is against you. But pregnancy rates for DI can be just as confusing as the "take home baby rates" offered by other purveyors of new birth technologies. A pregnancy rate of 70 percent is often reported, notes Sherman, and some will fail to note that this is after a year of treatments. "Almost all results have been expressed as overall success rates and only occasionally as cumulative rates, after a given number of cycles."[32] The cumulative pregnancy rate at the Sperm Bank of Northern California, for example, was 20 percent the first year of operation, 45 percent the second year, and 62 percent in 1983. But that was based on a woman going through one year of inseminations. Sixty-eight percent of all clients who start drop out for a variety of reasons.

Still, with older, more likely less fertile couples who are desperate for children, business is good for the holder of the stored sperm, the cryobank, and the doctor. Ninety-eight percent of the semen processed at Idant is shipped all over the United States, Canada, and South America. New York City males are providing sperm where religion makes it difficult to get—in South America, for example—and thus populating the rest of the world.

But the silence of the DI system of physicians and sperm banks has caused complex social and legal problems.

Lawyer Lori Andrews reports that "while doctors like to continue using donors of proven fertility, widespread use of a single donor in a limited geographical area could lead to unwitting incest of children of the same donor who grow up and marry each other. The possibility is remote, but in Tel Aviv, a marriage has already occurred between two DI children fathered by the same donor. In the United States, a similar marriage was stopped by a doctor who revealed to the couple their genetic link."[33]

A California doctor admits that he provided sperm for thirty-three pregnancies when he was a medical resident at Georgetown University in Washington, D.C., three decades ago. He now advises his children, all in their twenties, "Don't marry anyone from D.C."[34]

Barbara Raboy, administrator of the Sperm Bank of Northern California, formerly the Feminist Sperm Bank, tells of some places that operate with two donors for every fifty couples. At another, when one woman called for an appointment, the receptionist said, "Don't come in today. Your donor, John Smith, hasn't showed up." According to Raboy, "A common story you hear is that the doctor would promise [women] sperm, and they would wait and finally it was the doctor himself who was donating."

The Screening Issue

Many potential DI mothers are concerned about the lack of standards in an industry entrusted with the production of part of the future generation. Hillary worries about getting acquired immune deficiency syndrome (AIDS), and fears about that possibility evidently are not unfounded. Two Wisconsin women were reportedly inseminated with sperm from an AIDS victim in June 1987.[36] So far there is no indication that they have the AIDS antibodies, which would indicate infection with the virus.

Only a few of the twenty-three state laws regulating DI require that sperm banks conduct standard medical screenings of prospective donors. And most banks do not have the facilities to do background checks on the qualification of couples who request DI. The first client to give birth with sperm from the Repository for Germinal Choice in Del Mar, California—which advertises that its donors include geniuses and Nobel Prize winners—turned out to be a convicted felon who allegedly lost custody of her children from a previous marriage because of child abuse. No background check was done on the mother. "We have to rely on their honesty," said the Repository's spokesman, Paul Smith.[37]

Reproductive specialist Dr. Mary Hammond says, "The person in charge of our sperm bank, who is very concerned about the feelings of her donors, was very offended when we wanted to screen the donors and wanted to know why we were not screening the recipients, too. We have not been screening recipients either for gonorrhea or for . . . any of these things. We feel that it would just be too expensive."[38]

"Many people complain that the cattle industry does a far better job of screening donor bull sperm than sperm banks and physicians do," says Dr. Mark Perloe.[39]

In an attempt at self-regulation, the American Association of Tissue Banks (AATB), the trade association governing sperm banks, produced official guidelines for screening donors. The guidelines suggest tests for venereal disease, a family history to check for genetic defects, and setting clear criteria for rejection of donors. But membership in the group is purely voluntary and so are the guidelines, which do not apply to 80 percent of the inseminations in this country, which are done with fresh semen in a private physician's office.

"Spermatozoa and other cell tissues, and organs used in transplantation could legally and feasibly be regulated as a product subject to the jurisdiction of the FDA," notes Sherman, who fears that legislative regulations "may severely restrict or even eliminate cryobanking of human semen. Since 1976 there has been a close and watchful association between the FDA and the AATB . . . the FDA has taken the position that cryobanking and related transplantation have been adequately regulated on a voluntary basis through guidelines and education generated by the AATB."[40]

But, according to Andrews, "the majority of DI practitioners, apparently do not follow these standards." Andrews cites a 1979 University of Wisconsin study of 379 DI practitioners who were responsible for 3,576 births in 1977. "Although 96 percent took some form of family history from the donors, this 'history' often consisted of just asking the donor to indicate family health problems on a short list of common diseases."[41]

"I think the people who need the most supervision are private physicians," says Raboy, who has been associated with sperm banks since 1982. "A lot of people thought, it's the sperm banks who are bad. They're making a lot of money buying and selling sperm. . . . I do recognize that there have been a lot of problems with the banks, but there is nothing regulating private physicians."

For the consumers of sperm, it is apparently a "buyer beware" situation.

DI and the Law

Despite the long history of DI, laws governing the legal technicalities of giving birth to a child conceived of a donation lag behind practice, reflecting the gross ambiguity with which our culture views the practice. Like other procedures having to do with reproduction—abortion and surrogacy—we may half-heartedly condone it, but making it legal is another matter. In the 1950s, a bill introduced in the Ohio legislature but never made law suggested punishment for anyone involved with DI—a $500 fine and one to five years in prison.[42]

As late as 1983, twenty-seven states had no laws about sperm banks, making it unclear whether the husband or the donor was the legal father of the child.[43] In England, children conceived by DI are still technically "illegitimate," although no court has formally affirmed this.[44]

Many doctors routinely sign the "social" father's name to the birth certificate since, and according to Silber, that is apparently now the intent of laws in twenty-eight states. "Unless it is proved that the husband had no access to the wife, any child born of her is considered to be his by the law. Whether or not the husband is the true father, he is the legal father of any child born to his wife while they are living together."[45]

The legal questions posed by the tricky complications of the technologically simple procedure of donor insemination set the stage for the future ethical/legal questions of surrogate motherhood. Interestingly, if DI laws were applied to surrogacy, the surrogate's husband would be considered the legal father. Whereas the adopting mother in a surrogate situation must legally adopt the child, that is not a requirement for the father of a DI child.

The laws provide little guidance now, and until DI participants have occasion to challenge the law further—if there is the DI equivalent of a Baby M case, for example—we will continue to bestow fatherhood on the husband who resides in the house with the wife.

Anonymity

The policies of modern sperm banks and their physician mediators in the United States rest on a firm bedrock of anonymity, a protection that Boston law professor George Annas calls "almost obsessional."

This "protection" is manifested by an almost total lack of record-keeping. In fact, there are established methods of destroying records and deliberately obscuring lineage in this industry whose end product is a human being.

Idant, for example, isn't really sure how many babies it has sired. "Sometimes we don't find out until the couple wants a second child from the same donor that a first child was born [by]," says Feldshuh.

And usually the physician isn't keeping records, either.

"A physician in your town could do one hundred inseminations and not keep any records on them," notes Sherman.

According to a 1979 University of Wisconsin survey on DI, while 93 percent of doctors kept permanent records on recipients, only 37 percent kept permanent records on the children and only 30 percent kept any permanent records on donors. To further obscure the biological father's identity, almost one-third of the doctors used sperm from several donors during a single menstrual cycle. Most had no policy on how many pregnancies would be allowed from one donor. Further, 83 percent opposed any legislation that would require the keeping of records on donors.[46]

At Xytex, as at most sperm banks, the staff knows the donor but they don't know the recipient. Donors and recipients all are identified by number only, and, notes Karow, "All of our people are sworn to secrecy. It is fairly inconceivable that someone would find out." If a private physician does the insemination, he may know both donor and recipient, but he's not likely to be asked by one about the other or to volunteer much information.

Part of the reason for the well-entrenched anonymity has to do with protecting the social father from the heavy stigma of infertility. As long as he and his wife don't know the donor, he has no one to "upstage" him or to be envious of. Not knowing, in fact, is a kind of relief.

Dave, Martha's husband, briefly considered using his brother's sperm to inseminate Martha. Martha is vague about why this alternative ultimately did not appeal to him. Interestingly, the very idea of having the child of someone he *didn't* know seemed more acceptable than having the child of someone he knew well and who could provide a closer biological connection. She cited "lack of competition" as an important factor of influence.

"I talked to him about that," says Martha. "We didn't want to do that. I didn't ask him why. *He* really likes the idea of having this anonymous donor; he really does."

But it's not only the infertile husband who keeps the system working by the use of strangers. Anonymity has such a tight stronghold throughout the sperm distributing system that to remove it or even to jostle it makes all of the participants nervous. Everyone, it seems, likes not knowing.

"The most prominent and recurring theme among recipients and donors," notes Achilles, "is a disinterest in the unknown procreative partner. Among DI mothers this extends to uncertainty or lack of knowledge about record keeping and fear that they 'wouldn't like him' if they met him. Husbands of DI mothers are adamantly disinterested in the man whose sperm impregnated their wife. Donors express little interest in the recipient of their sperm, including a lack of concern about her marital status."

The donor's protectors, the sperm banks, say that donors would not come near a sperm bank if there were any hint that someone on the other end, i.e., the mother of their child or the child itself, knew who they were.

"The thought is that this [anonymity] is very important," says Sherman. "In general, anonymity must be maintained in order to have donors. In all the years, I've never seen a request to know who the donor is. They want to know the background and information concerning the donor, but not who. You wouldn't have a program without anonymity."

Australian Robyn Rowland's 1983 study of sixty-seven Australian donors found that 84 percent felt no relationship to the woman who became pregnant by them and 70 percent said they would *not* like to meet her; 22 percent said they would. Seventy-six percent were not interested in choosing recipients and 22 percent were.[48]

The Effect of Anonymity on the Offspring

There is growing recognition, however, spurred by the example of adoptive children who have demanded knowledge of their biological beginnings, that the "advantages" of DI anonymity on the part of the adult participants may be disastrous for the children. That to have a child (an act that would have required participation in the sexual act before donor insemination) by someone you don't know and don't wish to know has intense ramifications for the future generation.

"The anonymity between procreative partners facilitated by DI is an unprecedented social act," writes Achilles, who calls DI "a revolution in the reproductive process" with decidedly social implications.[49]

With increased attention now paid to genetic contributions to personality and health, some offspring—only those, of course, who know that they were conceived by other than one or both social parents—want to know the origins of their birth. Not having access to your other biological half can be a serious problem, considering inherited diseases such as Tay-Sachs, cystic fibrosis, diabetes, and sickle-cell anemia, as well as genetic predispositions toward heart disease and alcoholism.

"I think at some point our doctor destroys the [donor's] records," said a young Chicago mother of a DI child. "That disturbs us. We think maybe the doctor should keep some records [in case] there were cancer or heart disease, or the need for a bone marrow transplant . . . all the things you can think of. I would like to have access to that information. . . . But I don't really want him to have access to us. I don't want some stranger to show up someday, but I do want to know just the medical aspect."[50]

The idea of making sperm donation "open" conjures up a potential bundle of horrors.

"What if they started suing the father [donor] for child support," asks Dr. Antonio Scommengna, of Michael Reese Hospital in Chicago. "Or for tuition to send the kid to Harvard in twenty years? If the lawyers can find a way to get some cut from this thing, they will. No one in his right mind would want to donate without that anonymity."[51]

While Achilles notes that most donors want anonymity, a significant number may be open to the possibility of having their identity known. "Anonymous donors may be likely to feel anonymity is essential, and known donors are more likely to feel that knowing recipients is essential."[52]

If we are to acknowledge that sperm donors are human beings and not just DNA suppliers, we must also acknowledge that at least some of them may have thought about the end result of their action—a reflection that society encourages and demands when pregnancy occurs in the traditional manner and presumably to someone the biological father knows.

Sperm donor Robert says, "I would be curious as hell to see how they turned out. I hate to think that in fifteen years . . . someday I would be walking down the street and a twenty-year-old man walks by and we look into each other's eyes and I'd see a similarity."[53]

Although another donor George expressed "no interest in seeing these children," half of the donors in Achilles' study said they would be interested.[54]

Tom, a thirty-five-year-old divorced artist with two children from his first marriage, said, "Yes, oh yes, I think that's natural isn't it? I'd like to know what they look like, what they chose to do with their lives. It wouldn't bother me to be identified to that individual. I think it would be fair to them to look back at their genetic pool and be able to say, 'this is my heritage and this is what I can expect for my children.' "[55]

An "Open" Sperm Bank

When the Sperm Bank of Northern California opened in San Francisco in 1982, it began experimenting with the idea that donors would allow themselves to be identified when the offspring reached age eighteen, a practice that has been applied in Sweden for a number of years. Six months to a year later, the bank, originally founded as the Feminist Sperm Bank, enthusiastically offered what it called "identity release." With the donor's approval, the child eventually can know the identity of the donor.

Notes administrator Barbara Raboy, "We said, 'You're giving us a lot of information; would you be willing to have your identity released?' It was an interesting and challenging idea, but we weren't equipped to understand the consequences of that. We sat down with our lawyer and said, 'Could we offer something that could be protective of all the parties.' "

Now the Northern California bank is the only sperm bank in the country to offer the "approved donor the opportunity to have the sperm bank release his identity to the resulting child(ren), when the child turns eighteen years of age. This means that if a client conceives with a sample donated from a donor who has indicated 'yes' to identity release, the resulting child at or after the age of eighteen may contact the sperm bank to learn of the donor's identity. This does not imply that all parents will inform their child of this option or that all children will pursue the identifying information on the sperm donor.''

Unlike in other insemination programs where the doctor or staff does the choosing and the family is given little information about the donor, at the Sperm Bank of Northern California, recipients read from the same form the donor fills out.

Raboy says that 50 percent of the donors, 35 percent of whom are eighteen to twenty-four years old, are interested in the idea and do consent to their names being given when the child is older.

However, what a man does at age eighteen as an act of altruism, he may feel quite differently about later on. How can he decide that eighteen years from now it will be okay for a man or a woman to call him on the phone and say, "I am the product of your donation"?

In fact, sociologist Achilles finds that age may make the donor more reflective and more open to the idea. Just as many women who have abortions reflect seriously on it years later, men's reproductive activities may entail a delayed psychological reflex.

Barry, a donor, says, "At twenty or twenty-two, you don't think of anything—you just don't think that twenty years from now that you could have somebody out there. You just more or less do it and forget about it, and then three years later you think back about it.'' Barry, when asked if being a donor changed with the birth of his own child—"when I saw what my first son looked like . . . yeah."[56]

Says Achilles, "When you take the time and open some doors, you get the men to talk about their feelings, you don't just see them as donors. Most of these men would prefer to have their identity known, but they're not really sure what it will mean twenty years from now.''

Idant is "very much against" letting children know the donors. "We polled our donors seven years ago, and the majority would not be donors if they thought there was any attachment or responsibility. We make the distinction between a donor and a father. The father loves and cares for the child. The donor is a DNA provider. We don't even tell the donor if any semen is used or any children are born as a result. He has no attachment. . . . If you want a system with excellent donors with multiple characteristics, with intelligent, responsible people donating, they can't be subjected to something happening in twenty years. I even wonder, even if the person gave permission to be contacted in twenty years, in twenty years would he still feel that way? He has his own family—what are the ramifications?''

The ramifications of all new reproductive technologies are that there will be complexities not seen in a "normal" man-wife-child family. Like surrogate mothers who choose to bear children and give them away, donors who choose to donate their sperm to have children conceived of them should understand that their decision has far-reaching consequences. That is the nature of reproductive choices; the results go on to affect generations, even if the originators do not know about it. One solution to the anonymity problem affecting the resulting children might be the approach suggested by Dr. Cappy Rothman, director of the California Cryobank in Los Angeles, who destroys records but freezes a specimen of the donor's white cells for future genetic reference, claiming this eliminates any need to interfere with the donor's privacy.[57] But this continues the practice of anonymity in a system that is built on secrecy.

While Raboy, of the Sperm Bank of Northern California, recognizes the legal complexities of an "open" bank, she feels she must consider her responsibility to the offspring. "There is a big part of us that says, look, these guys are donors, all they're doing is giving part of their genetic material," she says. "But if the child wants to know, we have some responsibility there, too.''

Offspring: Opening Up

Candace Turner, the product of an artificial insemination, is in the manner of adopted children who yearn to know their biological roots, attempting to rattle the DI cage of anonymity.

If, as Dr. Silber says, "Patients are accepting it [DI] when there is no other solution, and many of the psychological, social, and legal fears about it are beginning to disappear," for others, the fears and psychological ramifications of a sanctioned institution are just beginning to hit home.

"I'm half someone my mother never met and would probably hate if she did," says the thirty-eight-year old Turner, mother of (she emphasizes) four "blood kin" children.

Turner's legal father, who had a vasectomy years earlier, was working in cattle reproduction in the late forties in Missouri. He and the mother decided what could work for cattle could work for them, and they asked the doctor to pick out some well-educated sperm, which eventually was used to inseminate Candace's mother and to produce Candace. At age thirteen, Candace was told of her origins. Now, after her marriage and the birth of four children, she has become heavily involved in a group she founded called "Donor's Offspring." Her stationery reads, "Unless handled correctly, artificial insemination can be a nightmare, not a panacea." Turner, like many other children of a donor insemination is also trying to find her biological father. Some of them call her, says Turner. These efforts are seen by sperm banks as an act of treason.

Turner feels that offspring have a right to know their other biological half. She cites the study of DI donors conducted by Dr. Robyn Rowland in Australia, in which 61 percent of the donors interviewed were willing to have their identity made known to their DI children once they had reached the age of eighteen and to have provision made for contact at that time.

The official policy of "Donor's Offspring" is that parents of donor-inseminated children plan to tell the truth at some point, probably before the children are of marriageable age.

In a system that has strategically and purposefully separated the sperm donor from his progeny, Turner is, against a strong tradition of anonymity, trying to put them back together. She hopes that in the future DI will be from a relative or husband. In such a case, the Birth Story will be altered to the degree the child looks like the husband. The child then can be told that several of the husband's male relatives donated sperm and that the lawyer or doctor picked one of the sperm. "Just tell the child that the identifying information is in a safe deposit box, in case anything should happen to you or until the child reaches the age of eighteen and wishes to know the name and see pictures of those to whom he or she is related."

Offspring—To Tell or Not to Tell

Hillary's child doesn't know and "we're not going to tell him," she says. "Sometimes I read articles talking about open DI and it unsettles me a little bit. Sometimes I wonder if he has the right to know . . . I don't know; it's confusing. He looks a lot like me and in a way he does resemble my husband. [The doctor] said the majority of the donors were medical students and we had medical students at the hospital [where she is a nurse] and I kept wondering [whether] it's one of these guys."

When her mother-in-law says, "Gosh, this doesn't look anything like Jack," Hillary cringes. "It doesn't upset him but it bothers me. I wish she wouldn't say that. I said, 'Do you think she knows?' and he says, 'of course not.' . . . We lied to her. She asked me point blank, 'Has he had a semen analysis and was it okay?' and I said, 'Yes.' "

Parents' confusion about whether to tell their DI children of their origins is understandable, given the pressure to pretend.

"A lot of the mothers don't tell anyone," says Achilles. "It's quite an incredible secret."

Even if parents have resolved the emotional complexities of DI between themselves, there is the ever present problem—the children. "I don't need to [know more about the donor]," says Martha. "But of course, you're always faced with the dilemma of what to tell your child. They say they want to have a look at the biological father. I think part of my anxiety was that I discussed this with people I probably shouldn't have; maybe one day my child would find out from someone besides us."

Most parents are told to continue the cycle of secrecy, to buy into the anonymity of the system.

"It is rather appalling that traditionally most doctors and lawyers who represent sperm bank clients have told people to lie," says Raboy. "The couple is advised not to tell the child for fear of undermining the social father."

Children may start to ask about their origins much earlier, but by age thirteen to sixteen almost every child is curious. There are ways to tell delicate things like this to a child. And there are ways not to tell.

One British woman, the product of insemination by donor, offers the way the news was told to her as a way not to tell:

"Mum decided that the truth must be revealed, for I was developing, would soon be a woman. She was too embarrassed, I suppose, to tell me herself, and she asked her lover of five years to explain the facts of my life to me. He asked if I knew about cows being 'injected' with test tubes of sperm; I said that of course I did, never being one to admit ignorance. There was obviously something more to all this, but I still did not predict what was to come next: 'That's the way your mum fell for you.' There must have been more questions from me and answers from him, but essentially I felt like escaping, carrying this great shattering boulder of information away with me. I had a picture of grunting farm animals, test tubes, sperm, and me. God the father had deserted me, I was the child of the devil—a pubescent melodrama that I acted out in hate and revenge."[58]

Again, there are ramifications of such knowledge of how one came about, and knowledge of the truth may strain relations as much, if not more than, secrets. Four of the five DI offspring contacted by researcher Rona Achilles mentioned spontaneously that they perceived themselves as smarter than their parents and attributed their perceived superior intelligence to their origins through DI. Tim, one of the children in the study, says that he feels "good about it because [he] knows [he] comes from a better selected gene stock than most others." That attitude, says Achilles, could be damaging to already strained relations within the family of a DI child.[59]

To tell a child is to acknowledge our culture's ambivalence about biological ties.

Achilles found that "a striking theme emerged concerning the social meaning attached to biological ties. Respondents expressed a dissonance on this theme, in some instances acknowledging and in other instances denying the social significance of biological ties. The defining social features of DI practice—anonymity between the sperm donor and recipients and secrecy about the procedure— testify to the social significance attached to biological ties."

On the one hand, biological ties are considered "virtually irrelevant. Donor insemination is described as something like an allergy shot or, more frequently, is equated with blood donation. On the other hand, biological ties are considered a significant component of identity and carry substantial cultural meaning," with the biological parents termed "real," "true," or "natural" parents. "If biological ties really were considered irrelevant, anonymity between the sperm donor and the recipient and secrecy about the procedure would not be necessary. Acquiring sperm, in other words, would not require the mediation, distance, and privacy provided by a physician."[60]

The people involved in DI have mixed feelings about biological ties, says Achilles—and how much they matter. To Achilles, these answers indicate "cultural confusion and uncertainty in comprehending and resolving the social consequences of donor insemination, particularly in relation to parental roles."

New reproductive technologies and new ways of forming and maintaining a family bring the heredity versus environment questions to an uncomfortable head—one for which we may not be prepared. If we comfort an adopted child with the solace that their "legal" father is more important than their biological father, if we say that genes don't really matter, why do we, on the other hand, invest so much in having a blood-related child by surrogacy, IVF, or DI? When we don't want genes to matter we conveniently say it is love that matters, but at other times we talk of blood—"You look like your father."

Achilles found that "biological ties have a lot of meaning in our culture and that it is important who the biological father is. We should be keeping records. We should be telling the children. Most of the children aren't told, or if they are told, it's under very poor circumstances."

After her baby was born, Martha still had to face fears about the donor and her child. She took a day off from teaching and took the baby to the babysitter. "I knew exactly what I had to work on. Part of it was a fear [that the donor would] harm our baby."

Martha and Dave who "look like brother and sister—we're kind of fortunate that way" have told their family but not most of their friends. Many friends will say how much their child resembles Dave. "It just goes to show that people see what they want to see."

Biological ties are so important that many couples will go to extraordinary lengths to conceive their "own" child, using scientific solutions—from fertility drugs to in vitro fertilization.

3

Infertility and the Great Hope of *In Vitro* Fertilization

"*In vitro* IS THE OUTER LIMITS," SAYS SUSAN CHAMBERS, THIRTY-seven, a lawyer in Washington, D.C. "You try everything before *in vitro*." She knows what she is talking about. For nine of the ten years Susan has been married to John, thirty-six, also a lawyer, they have done everything modern medicine has recommended to have a baby.

For Susan, a beautiful, slim, energetic woman, the quest has ended. In her spacious Washington, D.C., living room, baby clothes are stacked in chairs, there are flowers all over the house, and a banner above the dining room door reads: "Welcome Baby Riley." The Chambers have just held a large garden party to celebrate the arrival of a curly-haired boy who is being carried upstairs by the maid for his nap.

"It's been a long time," says Susan. "I was twenty-seven when we got married, and I was twenty-eight when we started trying."

Every morning for eight years, Susan has taken her basal body temperature and dutifully marked it down on a chart that she keeps in her bedside drawer—the chart tells her the optimal days to schedule sex. But that's the least of it.

When, after several months of trying she did not get pregnant,

Susan went to her gynecologist, who ordered a hysterosalpingogram to see if her tubes were open. So-called blocked tubes are a common cause of infertility in women. An estimated 600,000 women in the United States suffer from that condition. It can be caused by venereal disease, pelvic inflammatory disease (PID), which is sometimes brought on by an IUD, or by scar tissue from surgery and any number of pelvic infections. If the tubes are blocked, the monthly egg gets stranded on its way to the uterus and the man's sperm does not get a chance to fertilize it.

During the procedure, blue dye was sent through Susan's fallopian tubes and x-rayed. The dye flowed through the tubes into the abdomen. No blockage was revealed.

John was sent out for a sperm count.

"It was sperm of monumental proportions," Susan recalls with a laugh.

The doctor then decided that her problem was a tilted uterus and perhaps "hostile cervical mucus," a term that implies chemical warfare—too much acid—against the invading sperm. The doctor recommended a cream to neutralize the killer acid and having intercourse with Susan on her stomach.

"You can imagine! Here I have this gooky cream, intercourse on my stomach, and not getting up for half an hour so these little supersonic sperm don't have to swim against gravity. That was a real treat." Susan breaks into peals of laughter.

Desperate Hopes

One now elderly infertile woman with a tilted uterus recalls that she used to stand on her head for thirty minutes after sex because her doctor told her it would help her conceive. She never did get pregnant, and there is little evidence that a slight tilt one way or the other interferes with impregnation. But the myth survives, along with many other old wives' tales laced with well-meaning advice to struggling couples. It can be hard to deal with fertility tips that seem both insensitive and ignorant, but after a while most infertile couples learn to cope. Says one woman who has been trying to get pregnant for four years, "People say stupid things. A friend of mine has no tubes. When her old aunt told her to relax and she would get pregnant, she said, 'Gosh, that would be a miracle. I have no tubes.' It is more fun being totally honest. It makes them stop and say, 'I understand.' "

Even if infertile women get exasperated at advice counseling relaxation and romantic holidays, they are nevertheless likely to grasp at straws and fall back on tried, if not necessarily true ways of keeping hope alive. A few years back some barren women started to take the cough medicine Robitussin right before ovulation, not because they did not want any hiccups during intercourse but because it actually increases a woman's vaginal mucus. There were no reports about the effectiveness of Robitussin as a fertility drug, but if it might help, why not try it? Superstition runs rampant among the infertile. Although they may be hesitant to own up to it, hopeful women are likely to go to bed in a "lucky shirt" or bank on charms. Confessed one woman, "I'm almost ashamed to admit it, but I found myself with a stash of good luck charms during my infertility—several four-leaf clovers, a white elephant necklace, a red ribbon tied to my bed, a positive horoscope, and a Chinese fortune cookie that said my dreams would come true! Clearly my medical efforts weren't getting me anywhere, so I had to put my faith in something else."[1]

Susan's medical efforts were not getting her pregnant either, so after two years of gooky cream, she gave up on the doctor who had recommended it and went to a specialist.

Facing the fact that there may be serious problems is difficult for people who dream of starting a family.

Susan wanted both to experience pregnancy and to be a parent. "You know you're missing both of them," she says. "It is very difficult to understand before you have children how much of the hurt you feel is attributable to each one of them. It's just one undifferentiated pain."

A thirty-eight-year-old attorney whose husband also had problems says, "It was real devastating. You try for years not to have a baby, and then the irony of it is that you can't. There's an emptiness towards your whole life when you think you'll never have this baby. It's sort of an expectation you grow up with that you'll get married and that you'll have children. It's a basic premise of your life, and when it's pulled out from underneath you, it's hard to articulate what it's like. We both cried a lot."

A thirty-two-year-old woman who finally adopted a child admits "it was pretty rough. I would say for me the first overriding thing was major depression. Every time you see a pregnant woman, even if you were in a good mood that morning, within seconds you can go right down the basement. No matter what, it is always there. You just become absolutely obsessed with it."

Facing Fertile Friends

"We wanted kids so badly that we always thought we would," say Tim and Cindy, and they vividly remember the day they were diagnosed as infertile. "We came home from the doctor. It was our wedding anniversary, and my mother was having us over for an anniversary dinner. She had a priest come and say mass for us. He spent the entire homily talking about the children we were going to bear. We had just had terrible news, so we were very upset; we didn't want to tell anybody, so it was very painful. It is still etched in our minds."

To avoid painful situations, infertile people tend to isolate themselves. Some are ashamed of their condition and want to keep it a secret as long as possible; others simply cannot bear to be around people with children. Recalls one woman, "My most difficult experience was an evening spent with two other couples who had children. The children, their mothers, and I were sitting in the living room. One of my friends was rocking her newborn to sleep, while the other was playing with her toddlers. I sat in a corner of the room watching all of this interaction. It was almost dreamlike. I suddenly realized how out of place I was . . . a sore thumb. I felt such hurt, loneliness, and a terrible sense of emptiness. As usual, I held in my tears, and my friends never suspected my pain that night. But it is an evening I'll never forget."[2]

Sarah Peters, a professional woman from Pennsylvania, says, "I think the worst times were when my girl friends told me they were pregnant. It translated into our growing apart. Friendships became much more diffuse. They became much less close friends. They were preoccupied with their new children. It was socially isolating. It was a loss of a crucial social support system."

Says psychologist Susan Mikesell, "There isn't an infertile couple that hasn't talked about losing friends or feeling uncomfortable with friends. It's like all of a sudden you really feel like an outsider. They don't know how to deal with you, and you don't know how to deal with them."

Pressure for grandchildren can make a family gathering hell for those who are unable to produce them. Even when relatives are understanding and diplomatic, patience can wear thin. Says Cindy Connors, "We don't get a lot of support from family. They say things like: 'My God, you guys have been crying about this for four years. What do you mean, you're still upset about it? Can't you learn to deal with the situation?' But it is like a chronic illness. It doesn't go away, and you still deal with the different symptoms over and over again.''

"There are certain things that infertile people are going to find themselves experiencing that no one else they've ever known has experienced," explains therapist Constance Shapiro. "They tend to isolate themselves, and they don't have good support systems. They don't know that it is normal to feel jealousy when you see somebody nursing, that it's normal to feel anger when you get an insensitive remark thrown in your direction. In many cases their anger is justified—the anger they feel against physicians who are methodically plodding and slow, wasting a couple's time and money.''

Age and Infertility

Susan Chambers felt angry both with herself and her gynecologist for having wasted two years of her reproductive time. She knew as well as anybody that the older a woman gets the harder it is for her to get pregnant. She wished she had gotten to the fertility specialist much earlier.

More and more women delay childbirth until their career has been established and they are economically well prepared to support children. Susan, for one, finds it bitterly ironic that she chose to become a lawyer mainly to have financial security to offer the children who refused to arrive. Sarah Peters, forty-four, and her businessman husband, Steve, forty, were preoccupied with careers and, by their own admission, selfish. They also did not feel they were mature enough to have children until she hit thirty-nine, by which time her body was past its reproductive prime.

"The mean age of patients who come through our practice is thirty-seven," says Dr. Pierre Asmar, a fertility specialist in Annandale, Virginia. "I have fifteen patients who are in their forties. Most of them have no children." These are elderly ladies from a reproductive standpoint, who, if they do manage to get pregnant, run a higher risk of bearing children with defects.

Dr. Asmar recently gave a popular lecture about pregnancy over the age of thirty-five. "I couldn't believe the audience," he says. "Everybody looked over forty. We used to say no woman could have *in vitro* after thirty-five; now we cut off at, say, forty.''

Dr. Howard Jones, of the Jones Clinic in Norfolk, calls age "a major problem. We have become more and more occupied with people who are older, and this is partly because of postponement of childbearing—career women. Often there is a great deal of resentment that when they try to get pregnant they find they can't. They therefore blame heaven knows who, when, in fact, it was their own choice. A good many of them have found this very difficult to accept."

These "geriatric" would-be mothers keep fertility specialists busy. "From the age of thirty," says Dr. Michael DiMattina, a reproductive endocrinologist at Georgetown University Hospital, "there is a slight increase in the infertility rate simply as a function of age." His job is to counteract this rule of nature, and he recently did, making a woman very happy. "She was over forty," he says, "and she was up against tremendous odds because she had multiple problems. But we got a little luck on our side, a little technology, and we put it all together and now she's got twins."

Susan was hoping to find the winning combination of luck and technology when she went to the specialist. He started all over again with a complete fertility workup, listened to her medical history, did a number of blood tests, gave her a pelvic examination, and decided to do two endometrial biopsies, during which bits of the lining of the womb were removed and later examined under the microscope. The biopsies tell the doctor if the uterine lining is capable of supporting a pregnancy. The biopsies were Susan's "least favorite" part of the workup.

"They have to go through the cervix, and it hurt. Then they scrape some of the uterine lining off and your uterus starts to cramp up. They have to do two, so you can't kid yourself. The first time you're dumb, the second time you know," she says.

The Infertile's Knowledge of Reproduction

Like most women undergoing fertility treatments, Susan knows not only about endometrial biopsies but about every aspect of human procreation. If offspring depended on knowledge of the intricacies of the reproductive system, infertile couples would have hordes of children. They talk about the malfunctions of their bodies with an assurance and fluency that would put a medical student to shame. Without a stumble or hesitation, women drop terms like *hysterosalpingogram, laparoscopy, varicocelectomy,* terms that would choke a ventriloquist. Their familiarity with medical lingo comes from visiting doctors for years on end and from keeping up with fertility research published in the journals of medical and scientific associations. They not only read the stuff, they understand it. In their determination to find a way to have children, they often get one step ahead of the doctors.

"I've read everything there is to know about everything," says Susan. "You read to the saturation point. The doctors come in and say, 'Well, there is this and there is that.' 'Of course we know that! Don't you remember I asked you those nineteen million questions last time I saw you?' "

Fertility specialists have to keep on their toes. Dr. Mark Geier of Genetics Consultants in Maryland, an outfit that specializes in genetic screening, reports that patients will come to see him waving a publication and asking him if he has read it. Occasionally he hasn't, but he is not above swapping articles with his patients. These women learn a lot from their own misfortune, and they understand processes far more complicated than missile throw weights.

Any infertile couple can tell you that human life begins when a sperm meets an egg. A meeting between these two cells does not necessarily require an expensive dinner in a romantic restaurant and dancing till dawn in the moonlight, but it has traditionally required sexual intercourse. When a man ejaculates into a woman's vagina, he starts from 40 to 150 million kamikaze sperm on an elaborate journey that only one, or perhaps not even one, will survive.

While the lovers enjoy the afterglow of coitus—and perhaps a cigarette—the man's sperm are scrambling madly up the vaginal tract towards the cervix. But a lot of them will not even make it that far; millions die in the acidic fluids that keep the vagina clean. But the hardy ones will swim up the cervical canal within a few minutes.

The lovers may dose off without another thought to what is going on in the woman's body. Unless she is an infertile woman who keeps track of every step of her menstrual cycle with temperature charts, she might be alarmed to know that she is ovulating.

For about two weeks her pituitary gland, located at the base of her brain, has produced a follicle stimulating hormone, FSH, which encouraged growth in one of the circa 400,000 eggs housed in her ovaries. It also made the ovarian cells pump out estrogen, telling the thin lining of the uterus to start preparing for a possible pregnancy.

Once the egg has grown to maturity, the estrogen supply is shut off and another hormone, luteinizing hormone, or LH, orders the ripe egg to break through its blister-like casing, the follicle. The empty follicle, the corpus luteum, then starts producing the hormone progesterone, which prepares the uterine wall for implantation of the fertilized egg. The cells of the endometrium lining the uterine wall fill up with fluid, protein, and sugars to help maintain pregnancy.

Meanwhile, the egg, having left its follicle behind, has been caught by the fringe, the fimbria, of the fallopian tube that connects with the uterus. "The lining of the tube is like velvet. Millions of tall cells with soft hairlike tips called cilia brush the egg along in undulating waves towards the uterus. Cilia, mucus, and gentle muscular movements provide the sensitive ovum with a ride as smooth as a conveyor belt."[3]

While the egg floats in luxurious comfort, the sperm, like the brave knights of the Round Table, are being put through their trials. At the entrance to the cervix, the mucus plug that most of the time blocks the entry of both sperm and bacteria, has, during ovulation, changed to a clear and sticky elastic fluid that pours towards the vagina. Like salmon swimming upstream to spawn, the sperm have to struggle against the current in order to enter the cervix. It is also a struggle against time—the lifespan of the sperm is only about thirty-six hours. The sperm that were not overcome by either hostile or friendly mucus scramble on through the cervix and into the uterus on their way to the fallopian tubes.

The competition is still tough, many sperm and only one egg. The sperm are at a crossroads. There are two fallopian tubes and only a single egg, so one of the tubes is empty. Which way to go? Right or left? A lot of sperm make the wrong choice and rush headlong into the empty tube, where they eventually die. The rest are still in the race. They struggle against the cilia that carry the egg along but impede their progress; some get stranded in the little hollows in the tubes.

The lovers have gotten out of bed after a good night's sleep and have showered. He has shaved and she had put on her makeup. They look fresh and restored as they head off for work. The sperm meanwhile show wear and tear. The long journey has worn off the protective coating on the head of each sperm cell. By the time the sperm get halfway up the fallopian tube, they are completely bare-headed.

The dozen or so sperm that reach the egg throw themselves against it. It is still hard to get; the trials are not over yet. First a sperm cell has to penetrate the thick outer shell of the egg, and here more than brute force is required. It is essential to be first, for as soon as one succeeds the others stand no chance. The sperm cells bombard the egg with enzymes and one manages to make a little hole, only to discover an even tougher membrane underneath. More chemicals are released.

The lovers are totally unaware that a cataclysmic event is about to happen.

One sperm manages to get through the inner membrane of the egg. Sperm and egg fuse. Fertilization has taken place. (It can take anywhere from thirty-five minutes to thirty-six hours after intercourse to occur.)

Together as one, sperm and egg float on their honeymoon through the fallopian tube towards the uterus, and during the journey of a couple of days they divide first into two cells, then four and eight to become an embryo. The embryo now has a life of its own and is looking for a place to rest in the uterine wall, the endometrium, where after a few days it will implant itself and live happily for nine months. If it does not manage to attach itself, it goes out unnoticed the way the sperm came in, and all the trouble will have been for nothing. But in this case, the uterus is ready to receive the embryo, and before the couple know it, the woman is pregnant, or, as modern couples say, "we" are pregnant.

Timing is very important for conception. A man's sperm is in a state of readiness at any time of the month, but a woman's egg is ripe for fertilization for only a short period of approximately three days in every menstrual cycle.

Unlike other mammals, humans may feel sexual desire and copulate any time during the reproductive cycle, but unless intercourse happens to take place during ovulation, it is biologically for nought. In other mammals, desire and sexual intercourse are tied directly to the female's fertile period. There is no random copulation when the chances of conception are nil. A bitch, for example, can walk down the street without turning the heads of male dogs most of the year, but when she goes into heat, she is not only ovulating but emits an enchanting odor that attracts all the neighborhood male dogs and renders them senseless with desire. Dogs and other nonhuman mammals have evolved a system of procreation in which sex seems subservient to fertility, whereas among humans sexual pleasure appears to be almost an end in itself. It is only because human passions are so easily and frequently stirred that we manage to have intercourse during ovulation and to produce offspring as a result.

Judging by the high number of abortions in this country—one-third of all pregnancies in the United States were terminated in 1986—many people manage to get pregnant all too often. But, says Dr. Jeffrey Levitt, "Only if you're sixteen and in the back of a Chevy is it easy."

Human procreation is inherently chancey. For "normal" fertile couples there is only a 30 percent chance of getting pregnant per menstrual cycle, and some physicians put the odds even lower. Those who fail to achieve pregnancy within a year of trying are technically infertile. A lot of Americans fall into that category. Precise figures are hard to come by, but it is estimated that one in six couples—about 3.5 million couples—are infertile. Some projections are more pessimistic, and depending on the source, the quote for individuals ranges from 7 million to 15 million.

Surgery and Hormones to the Rescue

For Susan, getting pregnant was anything but easy. Despite having followed personal charts alerting her to the rise in her basal body temperature that means ovulation, her egg and John's sperm had not managed to rendezvous.

Susan's endometrial biopsies revealed a luteal phase defect—the endometrium did not develop properly at the right time. Pregnancy will not happen if progesterone has not made the uterine lining "wet and plush" and ready for the embryo. To correct that problem her doctor prescribed treatment with the hormone progesterone in suppository form.

"The suppositories look like candle wax, little bullet-shaped things," Susan explains. "They have to be kept cool so they don't melt down before use. Whenever I traveled on business I would have to get room service ice, and when I went to a friend's house they would have my progesterone in the refrigerator. It was really pretty funny."

Sarah Peters, who also went through so many treatments that she lost track, exclaims, "I forgot about the damn progesterone suppositories. Did I hate those! I hated the leaking. Argh! Of all the physical inconveniences of the whole process, what I hated the most was to take my temperature before I got up to pee, and second was the damn suppositories. I can take the pain of the shots and all that stuff a lot more than those two inconveniences.''

The progesterone might have done its job, but Susan still did not get pregnant. However her doctor had not yet run out of tricks. He wanted to see what was going on inside her and ordered a laparoscopy.

Laparoscopy is considered Band-Aid surgery because it requires only two small incisions that can be covered afterward with a small adhesive bandage, one in the navel and one just below the pubic hairline, but it has its ghoulish aspects. The patient is placed on the operating table with her feet in stirrups and is given general anesthesia. The patient is then tipped at a 45 degree angle with her head down and feet in the air, so that the force of gravity will make the intestines fall away from the pelvic organs. Her pelvic cavity is pumped full of carbon dioxide gas to push the abdominal wall away from the ovaries and uterus, giving the doctor a little ''elbow room.'' Introduced through the incision, the laparoscope, a bundle of quartz fibres that function both as a flashlight and a microscope, allows the physician to observe the state of things behind the abdominal wall. A probe is inserted through the lower incision so the physician can manipulate the organs.

For Susan, the general anesthesia was the worst part. ''I don't tolerate anesthesia well. I always think I'm going to die,'' she says.

Her medical struggle continued. Her doctor found that she had a mild case of endometriosis, a condition where errant bits of the uterine lining wander off and settle in places where they should not be. It is a very common condition and occurs with varying degrees of severity, and it often causes infertility. There may not be any outward symptoms, although pain during intercourse and severe menstrual cramps can be an indication. Some women are not aware of their prodigal endometrial tissue, which can spawn masses of foreign tissue on neighboring organs and require surgical re-moval. The condition can occur at any age but is most frequently seen in women over thirty who have never had children.

For Susan the doctor prescribed Danazol, a weak male hormone that suppresses ovulation completely. Without stimulation from the ovaries, the endometrium cannot develop and ''dries up,'' but the patient also becomes temporarily menopausal. The drug has a number of known side effects, from muscle cramps and lowering of the voice to personality changes, but Susan experienced only two: weight gain and hair growth.

"You have to shave your legs four times a day. You sort of have an evening shadow. It was ridiculous." She has a good laugh. "I hated it, I hated it, but mostly because of the weight gain. It was a big pain, and I had to take those pills every day for six months. On the other hand, you could rest emotionally. You knew you couldn't get pregnant, so you could have a normal life—except for the fact that you were fat and got gross, but at least there was not the constant 'Can you get pregnant?' "

Clomid and Pergonal: Tricking the Body to Reproduce

When the six months of Danazol were up, Susan had another round of dreaded anesthesia and laparoscopy to see if the Danazol had worked. It had, but still she did not get pregnant. Susan has lost track of chronology and the many drugs she was put on, but she remembers that she had fluid coming from her breast, which indicated a high prolactin level. Prolactin is a hormone that stimulates milk production in new mothers, and it inhibits ovulation. Stress may cause a temporary elevation of prolactin in the system, and, of course, infertile people live under chronic stress.

Susan's high prolactin level was brought down with the drug Parodel. "It didn't have much of a side effect, although initially I was nauseated for a while," she says, "but as long as I didn't throw up, I didn't care."

Still no pregnancy, so the doctor dipped into his arsenal of "magic bullets" and came up with Clomid and Pergonal.

If a woman does not ovulate properly, or even if she for unexplained reasons does not conceive, doctors are likely to try these so-called fertility drugs, which not only spur on ovulation but also correct luteal phase defects.

"Clomid," says Dr. Jeffrey Levitt, a fertility specialist in Maryland, "sort of fools the pituitary gland into producing more follicle stimulating hormone, FSH, so it makes the ovaries work harder. It feeds back to the system saying, 'Let's produce some FSH.' "

"Clomid is another wonderful drug!" says Susan sarcastically. "You have hot flashes. If you take Clomid in the winter, it is much better. On a ninety-degree day you feel you're going to fall out in the street because the heat inside is worse than the heat outside of the body. The daytime was hard to deal with, but the nighttime was even worse. It would wake me up."

For Sarah Peters, on the contrary, Clomid was "real nice. It made me feel sexier. It didn't last the whole time, but it was real nice."

If Clomid does not do the job, the patient graduates to Pergonal, an even more potent drug. It is a combination of luteinizing hormone and follicle stimulating hormone. These hormones are naturally and abundantly produced in the bodies of menopausal women when the system tries to save the faltering ovaries. The body is flooded with these hormones, and the excess is discarded through the urine. (This fact was discovered by an Italian biologist, Donini Serano, who decided to ask nice menopausal nuns to donate their urine to science. Today the Serano Pharmaceutical Company sends trucks around to Italian villages to collect the urine of elderly ladies in exchange for soap powder and other household items.[4])

"Pergonal," says Dr. Levitt, "supplies FSH and LH directly. It stimulates the ovaries directly. Pergonal can produce hyperstimulation and problems with that, and therefore you can put a person in the emergency room. Monitored properly, it should never happen, but maybe one or two percent of the patients might have a problem. Most of them can be operated on, but if you have multiple ovulation, basically you have an ovary that sort of explodes, so you must be very careful."

An even bigger problem with Pergonal is multiple births. Because the drug forces the ovaries into overproduction, instead of just one, several eggs are brought to maturity in one cycle. Twins are a fairly common side effect of Pergonal, and larger numbers are no surprise. With Pergonal there is one chance in 5,000 that the woman will have quintuplets. Without Pergonal the chance of that is one in 41 million. In the United States, Pergonal has produced thirteen sets of living quints and one set of sextuplets.[4] Since a woman's body is not designed for litters, multiple births are a mixed blessing, as one California couple, the Fustacis, will testify. Mrs. Fustaci gave birth to no less than seven babies, born twelve weeks prematurely. Four of them died soon after birth.

When Sarah, like Susan, went on Pergonal, she became anxious about taking "stuff that is associated with multiple births and big-time danger." But in spite of the severity of the potential side effects, "most women are willing to take the risk," says Dr. Stillman of George Washington University Hospital.

Pergonal is an extremely expensive therapy. "Fortunately, I could get it at a discount in price because I work in a hospital," says Sarah. "But it was still twenty-one dollars a package and I was taking . . . How many of those little suckers were we opening? Five or six packages an injection." And that's for five to seven days every cycle for six months usually.

According to Dr. Levitt, the normal price is $40-45 per ampule. Insurance may or may not pay for it.

Even though the drugs have proved safe for twenty-five years, continual hormonal stimulation may be hard on the body.

"With the hormonal stimulation we use," notes Norfolk's Dr. Howard Jones, "we think it's a good idea to let the body periodically cleanse itself. . . . What's the scientific evidence for that I'm not sure. I believe a little rest is just good for the soul. My own feeling is that it's psychologically better to take a vacation and come back and give it a shot than it is to keep at it all the time."

The Stress of Infertility

Why do infertile women put themselves through so much pain, fear, and emotional turmoil? Obviously to have a baby. But to people who do not want children or have them easily, barren women seem a bit crazy.

"Infertility is crazy-making," says Constance Shapiro. "Some of what we see as craziness in infertile couples I try to look at as a mourning response to the dream they have to give up. This dream is often bolstered by in-laws, friends, the entire social environment, baby showers, christenings, family engagements, little kids running all over the place. So it is hard for these people not to appear a little crazy to the normal fertile world, because they are trying to defend themselves against feelings of overwhelming grief, while at the same time carrying on the struggle which can take years." One author has called the pursuit of elusive babies "an all-consuming passion that burns up all other life aspirations."[5]

Struggling with failure after failure throws barren people into a state of self-doubt. And because they often suffer in isolation they begin to believe that they are both mentally and physically abnormal.

To help people share both their feelings and information about infertility, in 1973 Barbara Eck Menning established Resolve, a support group that now has chapters in many U.S. cities. Susan went to one of the meetings, asking herself, "What is an infertile person?"

"It is really funny, I thought these people have two heads. I was really nervous, kind of tense. I was really surprised when I got there. There were older people and younger people, black people and white people, professional people and nonprofessional people. It was just an enormous range of people."

Susan, though, did not become a regular member. Instead, she went to see a psychologist when she got to a state where, she says, "I would go into the baby department to buy a gift for a friend of mine and I would either feel I was going to throw up or burst into tears. I mean that's no way to live." Susan may not have started the sessions with the right foot forward. She told the psychologist: "I don't believe in this nonsense, but I can't survive this way, so if this will help, I'm going to try it." And Susan admits it did help having somebody to talk to about the ways inferility interferes with a "normal" life.

Sex and the Infertile Couple

A normal life implies a normal sex life, one that is not regulated by a temperature chart. Sex on schedule can take its toll. Kitty Sidler, a romance writer, and her husband, Loren, tried for four years to get pregnant and finally succeeded. Says Kitty, "One of the great things about being pregnant is that we don't have to have sex. Scheduled sex ruined our sex life completely. We had sex maybe a couple of times last year. We know we have to get started again. I'll look at Loren and I'll say, 'We have to have sex,' and he says, 'Oh, no.' We just don't want to face it."

Another woman told writer Linda Salzer about her difficulties. "The biggest problem was an absolute lack of desire. There was a lot of fantasizing. I would rather have been with anyone, including the milkman, than face sexual relations with my husband. It became boring, pressured, and so unspontaneous. It was like watching the Playboy Channel every night on TV—it just becomes repetitious. Plus the pressure to have to perform on certain nights was so uncomfortable. Monday night I might feel like it, but I knew that Tuesday was really the 'right night.' Then on Tuesday I would be nauseous and vomiting, but we had to have sex. I lived in Florida for many years and sex became like the weather there.

As pleasant as it is, you hate it after a while because you always know what to expect."[6]

For Susan and John it never got that bad, but, she says, "It is an awful situation to put people in. It really is. There is no real affection and there is so much pressure. After a while sex just becomes bizarre. John would want to make love at noontime. I would leave the office, and I didn't want to do it. I wanted to make love in the morning or in the evening, but at night he was too tired. Sometimes I felt I was on eggshells. I couldn't say this or I couldn't say that because it would destroy his mood. But I'm not a receptacle of sperm. Granted, I don't have to have an erection, but there is an emotional erection that women go through, too. You can't just jump into bed and say okay. It works both ways, buddy, although it is different physiologically."

Says her husband, John, "It becomes an annoyance more than anything else. You don't realize how annoying it is until you stop and don't have to worry about doing it on schedule. We both started to snap at each other because we both knew it was something we had to do, and neither of us felt like it. Sometimes it degenerated into an argument. There were a number of nights when we didn't do it."

Sarah Peters did not enjoy sex on schedule but, she says, "I'm astounded that Steve or any other man has been able to perform on demand on this timing business. It's amazing. I can't picture myself being able to do that. I'm impressed. It's a matter of true will, as far as I can tell."

It can be a source of great resentment if one partner is more conscientious about sticking to the schedule than the other. Some husbands do not like to perform stud service. One man complained to Dr. Joseph Bellina, author of *You Can Have a Baby*, "I can't do it like a machine. I had a really rotten day at work, and when I got home I just wanted to relax. My wife said, 'Hey, it's May 16.' I said, 'So what?' She didn't speak to me for a week after that." The wife felt her anger was justified. "It made me furious. I have tests, biopsies, a laparoscopy, all this stuff. All he has to do is have sex, and he wouldn't do it. How would you feel?"[7]

The Stress of Treatment

"One of the most difficult things about infertility and the whole process of going through these workups and all these programs and waiting month after month," Susan recalls, "is the incredible hope that you have that you'll get pregnant. You almost kind of will yourself. You just hope so much.''

Says one woman, who had surgery to correct her endometriosis and after four years finally did get pregnant, "There is always something in the back of your mind, you always think each month that comes along, 'Just maybe this month.' "

It is a constant emotional roller coaster, up from the time of ovulation and down to the depths of despair when menstruation begins. It is a terrible toll-taking strain on both husband and wife, but they react differently.

Says one struggling woman, "My husband, who didn't have a problem, was the stronger one and the listener. He would certainly bring it up, but usually it was me. His thing is that talking about it too much makes it worse; it's not going to make it any better. Sometimes it made me very angry, but in the long run it was helpful. After a while you do realize when you get so caught up in it you can't get away from it, that talking constantly about it doesn't make you feel better. So what I did eventually was to go to individual therapy because it was just wreaking havoc on me, it was upsetting him, and there really wasn't much he could do.''

"I was more cynical and pessimistic," says Susan. "That's what John would say I was. I was trying to be more realistic, and I considered his position overly optimistic, and that always worried me. I mean, he was optimistic the whole time, and sometimes I just wanted to shake him and say, 'Come down to reality now,' because when you're hit, you're really going to be hit. John is a very calm person.''

According to psychologist David Glass, "Often it is the husband who is out of touch with feelings and into denial. He will say to his wife, 'You're becoming obsessed with this and ruining our lives chasing all these options. We just have to relax and be calm and things will take care of themselves.' And the wife says, 'How can you be so out of touch with what is going on and unaware of my feelings? Don't you want kids?' '' I've seen lots of situations where the husband begins to believe that the wife is becoming psychotic; she appears obsessed and has emotional problems to the point where she cries every day. It becomes easy for her to believe that he is right, and she also becomes convinced that he doesn't want children, possibly because he doesn't care about her or about the marriage.''

Says Constance Shapiro, "The husband spends a tremendous amount of energy trying to perk up his wife a little bit. Often I find that, although men have feelings of sadness—and some of them are strong—they rarely let them come forth, because they have been so busy comforting and reassuring their wives. Because women are socialized to be more in touch with their feelings and to be open and straightforward about them, they let it hang out. Men who are not socialized to let those emotions out, tend to suppress them and be cheerer-uppers, although I'm not sure that men's feelings, when you really get at it, are so different."

John Chambers, in his guarded way, seems to agree: "I think there is a lack of sensitivity and understanding of what men are going through. I don't think people stop and think about the emotional wear and tear it can impose on a man, about how hard it is to go through a process like this."

Quite a few marriages have cracked under the strain of infertility, but those that survive tend to be stronger. Although their sex life has been ruined by the infertility—"It's rotten. We are not doing it anymore. It's gone."—Sarah and Steve Peters have become closer. "It really drew us together," says Sarah, "We were suffering together and we weren't blaming each other. I really think it forged us into more of a team with sensitivities for our joint experience. We had been kind of room mates before."

The Indignities of Infertility

Soon after Susan Chambers started with the fertility specialist, her husband, John, was asked to give a semen sample for a sperm count because a previous sperm analysis "was wacky." It turned out that his sperm count was not of monumental proportions, as the first count had indicated—quite the contrary. He had a low count and trouble with both motility and morphology, the speed and shape of the sperm.

The urologist, however, discovered a double varicocele on John's scrotum and suggested surgery.

Susan stayed with John on the day of his operation. When the doctor came in to check on his patient, Susan as usual asked her "million little questions." The doctor was finally on his way out the door, when Susan said, "Hey, wait. When can we have sex?" She burst into laughter at the recollection. "He kind of looks at the two of us and then he says, 'I don't think you'll feel like it tonight.' John was lying there stapled shut and totally doped up."

The surgery put John out of commission for about a week.

John's urologist gave him a fifty-fifty chance of being able to impregnate Susan after the varicocelectomy. To check the effectiveness of the operation, the fertility specialist wanted to do a postcoital test. Right around the time of ovulation, John and Susan had sex; she stayed in bed for about thirty minutes to give the sperm a chance to get into the cervical mucus, and then it was off to the doctor and up on the examination table, so the doctor could aspirate some mucus from the cervix and examine it.

The postcoital test was invented in 1869 by a New York physician, Dr. J. Marion Sims, who had an inquiring mind. The test was not well received by the scientific community, perhaps because Dr. Sims was conducting other, rather odd experiments, such as asking a man to have sex with his wife while she was under general anesthesia. (That experiment was designed to prove that a female orgasm was not necessary for conception.) It was not until a German doctor, Max Huhner, began to use it in 1913, that the postcoital test became part of the physician's standard repertoire.[8] Many infertile women probably wish that the test had been forgotten along with Dr. Sims.

"The doctors are intruding into something that is extremely personal," says Susan. "You know how personal lovemaking and family and all that is. I mean, you can't get any more personal than that. And then you have some guy cruising in the hospital and saying, 'Well, did you have sex this morning?' You just want to say. 'Give me a break. Don't I have any privacy?' And yet you accept it because you really want to have a baby."

Susan continues, "A lot of the stuff is—I don't want to say dehumanizing—but there are an enormous number of dehumanizing elements to it, and you struggle to hang on to your sense of self and dignity and humanity along the way."

As medical science and technology interfere in more and more natural functions, women become objects to be manipulated in the most invasive ways. To get through the dehumanizing and unpleasant procedures, they begin to look at their bodies as something separate from themselves.

"It is repeatedly subjecting yourself to indignities and invasions," says psychologist Glass. "That's where you see some of the detachment and denial that some women do in order to get through a procedure which is a turn-off emotionally. It takes its toll. A lot of women who have already gone through a lot get the feeling it's unfair that they should have to subject themselves to all of this."

"Infertility makes you feel like a lab animal," says Susan. "It really does."

Susan's mucus was examined under a microscope to see how many sperm were alive and well. Unfortunately, most of John's sperm were dead on arrival.

Resentments

Susan did not get pregnant, but John was still optimistic. "What I thought was: 'Oh, we have this problem, but it will take care of itself in time. It will be worked out.' You think that every time you go through a procedure." Susan's mood was different.

"John went to have this varicocelectomy, and that was fine, but I didn't think he followed stuff up enough," she says. "I was resentful because I couldn't even move out of one stage before I was into another stage. I was trying to anticipate and move ahead. If this doesn't work, what is next? But I don't think John was that way and it bothered me. We were going through everything and nothing was working. He finally went back to the urologist, and that was because I moaned and bitched. I had to push him hard to go back."

Because low sperm counts can be due to an insufficient amount of FSH in the blood, the urologist decided to stimulate John's sperm production with Clomid. Now both Susan and John were on fertility pills—Susan on her umpteenth drug, John on his first.

Clomid and Pergonal are "endogenously produced hormones," says Dr. Michael DiMattina of Georgetown University Hospital. "They are not synthesized by a company; they are naturally occurring substances."

"Well," says Susan, "the doctor says it's not a drug, it's a normal substance. Well, you don't naturally produce six eggs. It's not normal. *You* may call it a normal substance, but it is a drug to me."

Susan and John are not keen on pills. Susan even hesitates to take aspirin for a headache, but she says, "Our notion was, what difference does it make? If there is a possibility that it can help, you should do it if there are no major side effects.

"It is really amazing when I say it is no big deal to take a pill," she muses. "I'm a doctor's child, and I'm very anti-pill. You have to explain to me six ways coming and six ways going why I have to take this pill, because I'm not a normal pill-taker. So to go through all this medical stuff, to go through all this testing and all these procedures . . ." She seems to drift off into a silent survey of her medical history.

John did not get hot flashes, but Clomid did little for his sperm count either.

When Susan still did not get pregnant, her doctor suggested that they try intrauterine inseminations in order to save John's sperm the long journey through Susan's reproductive system.

John had to deliver this semen for months on end. "It gets to be ridiculous with all these tests and having to masturbate and run to the hospital, hoping you don't lose the sack on the way," he says. "It has to be kept warm, so you usually put it in your shirt pocket. It is in a little plastic sack closed with a rubber band. You get caught in traffic, finding a parking place. You worry about it leaking."

Intrauterine insemination differs from ordinary artificial insemination in two ways. The sperm is not left in the vagina but deposited right in the uterus, and the sperm is not used as it comes from the factory—it has to be "capacitated" first. The seminal fluid is washed away from the sperm, which are left to incubate for a few hours, during which time the protective membrane covering the head of the sperm self-destructs and makes the sperm ready to bombard the egg with enzymes.

"Sperm don't survive as well once you take them out of their natural media, but that's a problem of just timing ovulation," says Dr. Lanasa. "But again, it is only effective twenty-five to thirty percent of the time."

John's washed sperm was put in a catheter, introduced through Susan's cervix and deposited in the uterus.

"That was no fun either," says Susan. "Some days it would be marginally bad, some days it would be awful, awful, awful."

Susan went through a year of painful procedures, three times every month.

"I had gone through one of the intrauterine inseminations that was particularly painful, and I was upset," Susan recalls. "Damn it, I'm going through this; this is ridiculous, it hurts and for what? I was on the verge of tears. I said to the doctor, 'Please tell me when this is futile. Please let me know and don't let me go on if there is no use to it.' " The doctor promised, but her psychologist told her, "They will do those procedures on you until you're postmenopausal."

"I felt a certain amount of resentment as we went along," Susan admits. "I always felt that I was the one who had to have stuff done to me. Granted, he had the two- or three-hour or whatever surgery, and that's no fun, but I felt *I* was the one who schlepped to the doctor, *I* was the one who got the shots, *I* had to do intrauterine inseminations, not because I needed intrauterine inseminations but because his sperm couldn't swim, and that hurts."

Wives may begin to resent their husbands when their bodies are constantly put on the rack, and husbands may come to resent the physician, typically a male, even if he successfully induces pregnancy.

"Husbands are not overly fond of their wives' male gynecologist," notes Glass. "The more time wives spend seeing the gynecologist, the more there gets to be jealousy and resentment. It is as if the doctor is going to get her pregnant—and in a real sense he is—and the husband hasn't been able to, so husbands often get real fed up with their wives' trips to the doctor."

After years of infertility treatments—temperature charts, scheduled sex, pills, surgery, and undignified tests—neither Susan nor Sarah had conceived. Their hopes of getting pregnant the traditional way had dwindled. There seemed to be only one option left: external fertilization, or, in the popular parlance, test tube babies.

4

Test Tube Babies

IT WAS SIX YEARS AFTER THE BIRTH OF THE WORLD'S FIRST "TEST tube baby," Louise Brown, on July 25, 1978, that Susan and John Chambers decided to try external fertilization.

Louise Brown was the brain child to Dr. Robert Edwards and Dr. Patrick Steptoe. Numerous preliminary experiments on mice and women preceded the momentous event of her birth.

The Creation of the First Test Tube Baby

In June of 1963 Dr. Edwards, a British reproductive physiologist, mixed a sort of witch's brew of hormonal substances: "Take serum from a pregnant mare—this contained gonadotrophins— and inject it into an immature mouse; follow this up two days later with a drop of serum from a pregnant woman—more appropriate hormones in this human serum—and almost unbelievably vast numbers of eggs, not just a few, would hurry to ripen in the mouse ovary, sometimes as many as one hundred! If these immature mice with their overladen ovaries were allowed to mate with a full-blooded male, then dozens of embryos would be for the taking. . . ."[1]

Edwards got what he wanted: "Large mice, average mice, small mice—it was unbelievable—were all visibly pregnant," he wrote. "More than that, they were superbly pregnant, superlatively pregnant. Excited, we autopsied some of them immediately. There were fetuses everywhere. Gently we withdrew the uterus from the mass of intestines, kidneys, and other organs. Fetuses appeared from behind the liver, fetuses adjacent to the kidneys, fetuses tucked between the folds of the alimentary canal. One female carried thirty-seven baby mice, living and perfectly normal."[2]

For Edwards this was a particularly rewarding outcome of his experimentation. This was the "ovulation to order" he had been trying so hard to achieve ever since he had become bored with his initial studies in wheat, oats, and barley at the University of Bangor in North Wales. Animal genetics was much more exciting, especially when, as he had done now, he could control ovulation. In the genetics lab at Mill Hill in Edinburgh, where Edwards was working at the time of these experiments, he found he could have eggs whenever he wanted.

There were "other exciting prospects: What about affecting super ovulation in farm animals? How valuable that might be! And what about human beings? Those women who had difficulty in having children—could they be helped?"[3]

Edwards thought that if he could get human eggs, he could concoct a culture recipe that might help ripen the eggs outside the body—a little salt, a little potassium chloride, glucose, a touch of protein.

He was making progress. He planned to write up his discovery for a scientific journal but became disheartened when a review of the literature revealed that an American, Gregory Pincus, developer of the contraceptive pill, had already succeeded in ripening rabbit eggs in a culture solution.

But Edwards persisted, seeking to duplicate with human eggs what Pincus had done with rabbit eggs. His main obstacle was one of egg supply. His work demanded a large supply of human eggs to experiment on, and the only way to get them was from human ovarian tissue removed "for medical reasons." He explained his needs to the gynecologist who had delivered his own child at the Edgware General Hospital. The gynecologist agreed to help. Before operating on a woman, usually to perform a hysterectomy, the gynecologist would phone Edwards "if any possibility arose of a small piece of ovarian tissue becoming available." Standing by in the operating room, Edwards would come forward at the appropriate time "clutching my glass sterile pot—the receptacle for the precious bit of superfluous ovarian tissue."[4]

But the jump from mice to men was difficult. Mouse eggs ripened in two hours, but human eggs just sat there. Three, six, nine, and twelve hours later nothing had changed. Edwards was frustrated, sure that Pincus had been wrong. Finally, when he looked at the eggs after twenty-eight hours, he was delighted to find that "the chromosomes were just beginning their march through the center of the egg."[5]

Keeping a steady supply of human eggs was a continuing problem. Explanations to doctors that the future solution to problems of infertility lay in these experiments fell on deaf ears. When Edwards' egg source dried up, so did his research. He moved to Cambridge University, where he was able to get monkey eggs, sheep eggs, and cow eggs from a nearby slaughter house, but it was human oocytes that he really needed.

Finally managing to obtain three of the rare human eggs and getting them to ripen, he decided to try to fertilize them with his own sperm. Nobody thought it would work; the belief at the time was that spermatozoa needed to be in contact with the secretions of the female reproductive tract. But when Edwards returned to the lab, he found that one sperm has passed through the membrane of an egg. Sperm and egg had not completely fused, but the fact of penetration was encouraging.

Edwards' egg deficiency problem was solved by professors Howard and Georgeanna Jones, researchers at Johns Hopkins University in Baltimore. Edwards went to work with them at Johns Hopkins, funded by a Ford Foundation grant.

In July 1965, the first time Edwards met the Joneses, they agreed to help with his experiments. "I was to share pieces of ovarian tissue with the pathologist and my work started within a week."[6] Happily surrounded by plenty of ovarian tissue, it occurred to Edwards that perhaps sperm that had resided inside the cervix might somehow be a more potent fertilizer. Edwards and Jones collected spermatozoa from the cervix of patients soon after the patients had had sexual intercourse, but this proved ineffective, too.

Upon his return to Cambridge, where only animal eggs were available, Edwards was again offered help by Americans promising the opportunity to work on human eggs, this time at Chapel Hill, North Carolina. There Edwards tried to "incubate" sperm in women's wombs before using it to fertilize the eggs. He made a "small chamber" lined with a porous membrane that would allow uterine secretions to pass into it but not out, filled it with sperm, and inserted it into the wombs of volunteers.

"What business it all was: collecting pieces of human ovarian tissue, ripening the eggs, collecting spermatozoa and putting them into little chambers, and then finding a volunteer who would allow this chamber to be inserted into her womb. I have cause to be grateful to those ladies of Chapel Hill who volunteered in sufficient numbers for me to continue my research. The chamber with its busy spermatozoa would be inserted at night and removed the next morning, and I must confess that I had many a sleepless night fearing the chamber would burst inside the uterus, releasing the spermatozoa with disastrous results. . . . Fortunately the membrane held," wrote Edwards.[7] But the sperm did not perform any better after this treatment.

Edwards met the other half of what was to become the test tube baby team in the fall of 1976. He had read about Dr. Patrick Steptoe's ability to collect eggs from the fallopian tubes through a laparoscope. Steptoe was working at Oldham General Hospital, three hours by car from Cambridge, and a hospital not well equipped for research.

Steptoe, a gynecologist, had done a number of laparotomies during which he had to open up the abdominal cavity sometimes purely for diagnostic reasons and wished for a safe and efficient means to peer into the abdomen without having to resort to laparotomy. He learned that a doctor in Paris was working with an instrument called the laparoscope, a telescope-like device with an eyepiece to look through and a lens permitting the physician to look inside the abdomen when the instrument was inserted through a small incision in the abdomen. He acquired one and began to practice on fresh cadavers. Once he'd learned to use the device, he began to employ the laparoscope for diagnosis and treatment of patients.

With the laparoscope, Steptoe explored the fallopian tubes and obtained tissue specimens. If sperm could be introduced this way, he thought, a woman could get pregnant. (He used the laparoscope for sterilization as well, destroying a small piece of each fallopian tube with an electric current. This is now a common method of surgical birth control.)

Edwards and Steptoe started working together on April Fool's Day 1968. Steptoe routinely explained to patients admitted for hysterectomies that they should have intercourse with their husbands before the operation, so he could collect sperm from their fallopian tubes. Meanwhile, Edwards, with the help of an assistant, had figured out a new culture that would capacitate the sperm. It contained an energy source, a few salts, a protein extracted from cow serum, and penicillin. The new culture worked, so he no longer needed sperm collected from a woman's body.

In March 1968 a gynecologist friend provided Edwards with ovarian tissue from which he retrieved twelve eggs. He fertilized them himself and put them in the culture. Ten hours later "some ova were in the early stages of fertilization with the sperm tails following the sperm heads into the depths of the egg."[8]

Their story broke in the British journal *Nature* in 1969. "Life is Created in Test Tube" read the headline over the article. The negative reaction of the popular press to these "immoral experiments on the unborn" did not stop Edwards and Steptoe.

Nineteen seventy-one, however, was a hard year. Edwards and Steptoe did not get any funding for their research, fertilizations did not work well, and they discovered that the fertility drugs they had prescribed for the infertile women they were experimenting on shortened the menstrual cycle, so that by the time they had collected the eggs, fertilized them, and let them grow to the eight-cell blastocyst stage, the womb was preparing to shed its lining—to menstruate. They toyed with the idea of freezing the embryos and implanting them during the next cycle, but none of the frozen embryos proved capable of growth. They also worried about moral and legal issues.

Once they got reliable fertilization and embryos, the problem was to pinpoint the best time of removing the eggs. A new urine test that indicated the level of luteinizing hormone in the body helped them. But why wouldn't the transferred embryo stick to the uterine wall?

Several women had already left Oldham Hospital disappointed when Lesley Brown, age twenty-nine, came to Dr. Steptoe in the fall of 1976. She had wanted a child for ten years, but her fallopian tubes were blocked. She was desperate. Her marriage was breaking down because of her infertility.

Steptoe performed a diagnostic laparoscopy and decided an operation was necessary to clear away adhesions and to remove the diseased tubes.

After recovery from the operation, Lesley Brown was ready for the *in vitro* procedure, but Edwards and Steptoe still were not sure exactly when to harvest the egg. "Would we be able to time it just before the follicle ruptured and released the mature egg into the abdomen, where it would be lost irrevocably? Even if Bob could solve this timing problem, it would mean that I and all my team would be tied to the patient's menstrual and ovulation cycles," Edward wrote.[9]

Using the new urine analysis, the doctors tested Lesley's LH level every few hours, and twenty-six hours after they identified the onset of her LH surge, they prepared her for laparoscopy. Her husband, John, was there ready with a fresh semen sample. The semen was centrifuged and prepared while Lesley was on the operating table. Steptoe inserted the needle, found the ripe follicle, and withdrew the egg. The egg was placed in a petri dish with the sperm and the waiting game began. By evening fertilization had taken place, but the egg still had to divide into eight cells before it could be implanted.

Thirty-six hours later "it was beautiful: eight rounded, perfect cells." The embryo was placed back in Lesley Brown.

On July 25, 1978, the term *test tube baby* was applied to seven pound, two-ounce Louise Brown, extracted by cesarean section from her mother's abdomen, innocent of her role in the evolution of mankind's meddling with the universe, but a crowning glory to Edwards' and Steptoe's experimentations. An egg and a sperm united in a petri dish outside the mother's body had grown into a normal baby.

Clifford Grobstein, professor at the University of California–San Diego and author of *From Chance to Purpose*, compared the achievement of Louise Brown's birth to man's landing on the moon in 1969. Now man had conquered "inner space" as well. There was new hope for the battalions of infertile people.[18]

The Numbers Game

About a year after Louise Brown opened a new era in reproduction and started serious debates on the moral, legal, and medical implications of the methods used to bring her into this world, another baby girl was born in obscurity in America. She was conceived when her mother, Cindy, a college student, had a weekend fling with her old boyfriend. Immediately after her birth, the baby was given up for adoption.

A few years later, Cindy married Tim Connors, a college student in his senior year. They decided to start a family. Having conceived all to easily the first time, Cindy was expecting to have a baby soon after Tim's graduation. They celebrated graduation, but months ticked by without a pregnancy. Suspecting that something was wrong, the Connors consulted a fertility specialist, who gave them terrible and surprising news: Tim had a low sperm count and Cindy had blocked tubes. The usual regimen of scheduled sex, regular visits to the doctor's office, and several surgeries to open Cindy's tubes took over their lives, but it was all to no avail. No baby. Finally there was only one solution left: *in vitro* fertilization.

"I was very scared," says Cindy. "It was scary to make the decision to do it. Part of it was that *in vitro* is the last step. There is nothing we can do afterwards, and we didn't really want to admit to ourselves we were at that point. It is very hard to let go. I don't think we were scared of the *in vitro* process; we had been through so much—what was one more procedure?"

Even under normal circumstances human reproduction is chancey at best. For fertile couples who want children and have no problems, the average time is 5.3 months to get pregnant, says Dr. Jeffrey Levitt an infertility specialist in Maryland. Although some IVF programs boast that they can do better than nature, the opposite is actually the case.

The success rate for IVF has been climbing steadily, but the numbers are still rather dismal. The pacesetter in this country is the Jones Clinic in Norfolk, Virginia, where patients in the *in vitro* program have about a 20 percent chance of getting pregnant.

"The odds are so poor," says psychologist Susan Mikesell. "But when there is so much stress around it, your objectivity disappears. So when you hear there's a ten percent or twenty percent chance of coming away with a live birth after the procedure, you don't look at it as an eighty percent chance of not getting pregnant."

And even those numbers can be misleading.

"It is not one out of ten people who walk in the door, or even one out of ten who is evaluated and accepted into the program," says psychologist David Glass. "It is not even one of ten who starts the cycle; it's more like one out of ten who starts a successful cycle where they have retrieved a certain number of eggs that have fertilized. That person will be one out of seven or whatever."

For every patient who has one or more embryos transferred in a particular treatment cycle at Norfolk, for example, the chances of pregnancy are 27 to 31 percent, but that does not take into account women whose eggs were not retrieved, whose eggs were collected but not fertilized, etc. Another way of looking at it, says Norfolk's director of research Dr. Gary Hodgen, is that "for this program, for each cycle of treatment, about twenty-two babies will be born for each hundred treatment cycles."

With the short numbers in mind, one woman who had gone through an operation for endometriosis and various other treatments and still did not get pregnant chose to stop the baby chase before *in vitro*. "I just couldn't get myself psyched up for it. I just couldn't. And when you do IVF, you've got to believe it is really going to work."

Impossible odds did not deter Sarah Peters, who at forty years plus, had no time to lose. She had failed to conceive after treatment with Clomid and Pergonal, but she was optimistic about IVF even though her chances were terrible.

"You want to hear odds?" she asks. "I have fibroid tumors and a little bit of endometriosis, so even if it worked, there would be a forty percent chance of spontaneous abortion. If you add it in with the something like twenty percent chance of the embryo taking, it comes down to a three percent chance that a kid could come out of it alive, and I was still willing to do it."

Caren Ellis, a thirty-eight-year-old lawyer, had also come to the end of the line after having her tubes tested, after two endometrial biopsies, and after Clomid and Pergonal. She was not too keen on *in vitro*, "but my husband really wanted to do it," she says. "This was several years ago, and there weren't too many programs, and those there were, weren't too successful. But the doctors were saying, 'If it were my wife, I would go to Norfolk,' so we went down to Norfolk."

Procreating at Norfolk

The day Louise Brown was born in England, Howard and Georgeanna Jones were moving into their new house in Norfolk, Virginia. Having had distinguished careers as gynecologists at Johns Hopkins University, both had been invited to serve at the Eastern Virginia Medical School.

When a Norfolk newspaper reporter, seeking a reaction to news of Louise Browns's birth, asked Howard Jones, an early collaborator of Edwards', if he would have an *in vitro* clinic at Norfolk, Jones offhandedly answered that they would—if they could find the money to get started. Only days later, a grateful patient of Georgeanna's who had had a baby with medical help, called to say that she would contribute $5,000 to get the program going.

By 1979 the Joneses had applied for a "certificate of need" from the Eastern Virginia Health Systems Agency in order to start a program for "Vital Initiation of Pregnancy." They also applied to the Department of Health, Education, and Welfare for $200,000 in research money, to do what Howard Jones calls "just an extension of what he had been doing for a number of years, namely, helping people who had a problem. This was a new opportunity, a new method of approaching it."

Later that year, having heard about plans to perform what many still consider highly controversial manipulation of the private recesses of the body, the local public opened discussion on whether they wanted test tube babies in their back yard. On Halloween night, October 1979, several hundred people met for a public outcry at the Norfolk Public Health Department to protest messing with the earliest and most vulnerable stages of human life.

Howard Jones, codirector now of the Howard and Georgeanna Jones Institute for Reproductive Medicine, says that the protest was "largely led by the Right to Life group, which is no specific group, composed of religious people of various denominations, and I think a good bit of that was triggered by ignorance of what it was really all about."

Protesters were concerned, recalls Jones, that IVF children would not be normal, and "there were trivial sorts of silly things—like I remember one woman said this would be like—what did she call it?—'adultery in a dish.' It's silly, and there were a lot of other arguments of that sort of trivial nature that really, I think, did harm to the cause that they were trying to promote because it was so apparently not thought through."

Still the Joneses were worried that their plans might be obstructed.

"We were concerned that there would be political issues involved. The individual who ultimately had to make the decision was a government appointee, and government appointees of elected officials are greatly influenced by the noise that people make."

Nevertheless, five months after the hearings, the Joneses won. On January 25, 1980, the Norfolk General Hospital received approval to go ahead with their plans for a fertility clinic, and in April 1981, Judith Carr, the thirty-fifth woman to go through the program, became pregnant with an egg and a sperm that had met in a petri dish at the Norfolk clinic.

News of the success spread quickly, and the Joneses were soon bombarded with requests for treatment by infertile people from all over the country.

"I remember my first time going in there," says Caren Ellis. "I was really so excited. It was so glamorous. There were about twenty women sitting there chatting. You felt kind of like an outsider in a big family, and all of a sudden I thought, 'Oh gosh, I don't think I want to be here. It doesn't look like a whole lot of fun.' "

Judging by the deadpan way Caren recounts her experiences at Norfolk, it is no fun at all. It sounds a bit like boot camp.

Located on the sixth floor of Hofheimer Hall at the Eastern Virginia Medical College in Norfolk, the Jones Clinic looks like any other waiting room. Tastefully done in pale blues, the room is busy twice a day: at 7:00 A.M., when blood tests are done, and at 4:00 P.M., when the results come back. The phone rings incessantly. A fat scrap book covered in red gingham and bordered with white lace shows the happy end products of the egg transfers done across the street in Norfolk General Hospital.

In an adjoining conference room, there are pictures of the new facility the Joneses hope to build, and a sign:

> The Norfolk group is the acknowledged leader in IVF and embryo transfer in the United States. This, with the fact that theirs is the unit that has been at it the longest in the field in this country (established 1980), make their leadership an uncontested fact.
> —*New England Journal of Medicine,* April 9, 1987

The room is full of men and women who look to be in their thirties.

"I have to go now to the transfer," says one woman to her husband, and she disappears behind the door.

This is series number 28—one of the eight-and-a-half-week cycles during which the staff works seven days a week, their lives revolving around a kind of gamble on ovulation. Every eight and a half weeks, they take three or four weeks off. There are five series a year, treating 800 to 1,000 couples a year.

There are counselors with baby pictures on the walls. There are doctors with white coats and proud faces when a success comes back to show them their baby.

Sometimes in this area, says the clinic PR director, pointing to a small foyer secluded from the offices and waiting room, couples get the bad news. "Here you see people who are unhappy," she says. "So this gives them a little chance to readjust before they go back out into the waiting room."

The Steps of IVF

"We're making the assumption from the start that [the women who come here] are very anxious to do it," says Jones, "that they have considered all their options and that they're here to get in the ball game."

The patients report on the morning of day three of their menstrual cycle. After an orientation, blood is drawn. The next day, the women get shots of Pergonal, one in the morning and one in the afternoon, to stimulate the ovaries into overproduction. The recruits, organized into numbered series, set up camp in a nearby hotel, where they stay until the embryo transfer takes or until they drop out. They have to be at hand for daily blood tests and hormone injections.

"Most everybody complains of being tired from the shots, and more emotional," says Caren. "I put on some weight, but that could just be the stress. You eat more because you feel like treating yourself because you have to go through this." In order for the physicians to monitor the hormone levels accurately, the hopeful-mother brigade has blood drawn first thing in the morning at 7:00 A.M.

"It is so tedious to have to go in every morning to have your blood drawn and get your shot and stand around in line with twenty-odd women all anxious to get out of there," remarks Caren.

Checking the Follicles

On day six the doctors start doing sonograms of the follicles to see if they are developing properly. Sound waves are bounced off the tissues to be examined and are transmitted as visual images on a television screen. The doctor will get a clearer picture if the sound waves travel through water rather than air, so the patient is asked to drink six to eight eight-ounce glasses of water to fill up her bladder before the examination. With her bladder full and her bowel empty the patient lies on the table and has mineral oil rubbed on her stomach to allow a cursor to glide over her skin and transmit images of her interior. The follicles appear as dark circles on the monitor. The bigger they are, the closer they are to ovulation.

Sarah Peters, who went through a similar program in Pennsylvania, remembers the discomfort of a full bladder. Not surprisingly, "it feels like you have to go to the bathroom real bad and somebody is pushing on your bladder," she says. "I have seen women act up outrageously with the discomfort. Until you get used to it, it's uncomfortable and unpleasant, but, God knows, it's not as bad as losing a limb."

Sonograms are not just a one-time occurrence.

"It turned out half the month I was in there in the morning for a sonogram," says Sarah. "You had to do a baseline, and when you could possibly be ready, they started to time the size of the follicles every day. It came out to be a half-time job."

The doctors also do pelvic exams to see if the cervical mucus has changed to an elastic fluid, which means that ovulation is near.

The daily blood test, which monitors a rising estrogen level; large follicles, fourteen to fifteen millimeters in diameter; cervical mucus; and urine tests showing the amount of luteinizing hormone in the body, all help to pinpoint the time when the patient will be ready for the egg retrieval.

Because Pergonal completely short-circuits the hormonal system, a day or two before the eggs are to be removed, all the women get a shot of HCG, human chorionic gonadotropin, a hormone that closely resembles luteinizing hormone, in order to mimic nature's signal to the ovaries to gear up for ovulation.

"You have thirty-six hours notice before harvest," says Jones. "With the method currently in use, the egg will not complete its final maturation, so you have to have something to do that—HCG. And it gives the husband time to get here."

The eggs to be harvested have to be ripe or they cannot be fertilized, but they must be retrieved before they break through the follicles. If the eggs are released before the doctor can get to them, as occasionally happens, they disappear forever into the blocked ovaries or the abdominal cavity.

"You know, you can go through the whole thing, and if you ovulate, the whole thing goes down the drain. Then people get sent home, and that adds to the stress and anxiety," says Caren.

Nan Tilton, the first American woman to have *in vitro* twins, described the level of anxiety among the women in the Norfolk program: "When the women got together, they never talked about anything but *in vitro*—who had gone for surgery, how many eggs did she have, how many were transferred, who was sent home, who was getting FSH, who wasn't, whose husbands were staying. . . . We were all at the verge of hysteria, our hormones were going wild. There was the tension of waiting and not knowing what was happening. Here we were sitting around doing nothing because that's what we were supposed to be doing, while the doctors manipulated our bodies to make them pregnant."[10]

"Sometimes the doctors weren't real sympathetic," says Caren. "They kind of made you feel you were just another body. You feel you're just being run through the mill."

The Egg Retrieval

The next step for those who have not been sent home is the actual egg retrieval, usually on cycle day eleven. The husbands are at hand to supply semen to fertilize the harvested eggs.

The egg harvest takes about half an hour.

While the patient is under general anesthesia, two incisions are made in the abdomen. The physician can see the follicles through the laparoscope, and, using a hollow needle, he punctures the ripe ones and aspirates the eggs. The chances of getting an egg are better than 90 percent, says Jones, and "when you don't, it's in a way predictable; it's usually the fringe patients—forty-two years old and won't take no for an answer." Each egg is assigned a number and taken to the lab.

Lab technicians examine the eggs. Occasionally an egg is over-ripe and has to be discarded. The eggs with potential are incubated at body temperature for about six hours, and those that are slightly immature are given a longer time to ripen.

The incisions are stitched up and covered with Band Aids, and the patient, after a shot of antibiotics, is moved to the recovery room, where she stays for several hours until the anesthesia has worn off.

Caren was barely out of surgery before she asked, "How many eggs did you get?"

The more eggs there are to fertilize, the more chances that one will end up as a baby.

In the early days of *in vitro*, it was unusual to get more than two or three eggs, but advances in the administration of hormones have made a much larger number common. In Dr. Jane Chihal's Dallas infertility clinic, the average number of eggs harvested is five to six. There is, of course, no guarantee that all the eggs will fertilize, but doctors have become so good at creating embryos that a couple often end up with more than is safe to transfer back into the uterus. Dr. Chihal never puts back more than three embryos; many other clinics set the limit at four. Although all the embryos rarely take, there is always the danger of multiple gestations.

Joining Egg and Sperm

When the woman goes into surgery, her husband is given two small containers and asked to produce a semen specimen, one a few hours after the laparoscopy and another twenty-four hours later in case immature eggs have ripened. The semen sample has to be kept at body temperature, and it must be at the lab within thirty minutes of ejaculation. There it is capacitated for its petri dish rendezvous with the wife's eggs.

While the sperm and egg get together and begin to divide in their hormonal solution, the patient goes back to the hotel to recuperate. If the sperm succeeds in fertilizing the egg, the resulting zygote stays in the petri dish until it has divided into an eight-celled embryo and is ready to be transferred to the woman's uterus, usually about forty-eight hours after the retrieval.

"We were so nervous thinking about our eggs over there all alone in the laboratory, wondering if they were fertilizing," Nan Tilton recalls. When, the day after laparoscopy, the Tiltons ran into a doctor at the clinic and asked for news of their eggs, they were told, "You're not supposed to be here . . . We have a thousand eggs over there in the lab to look at. We don't have time to talk to everyone who comes around asking about theirs. Go back to your hotel room and wait for a telephone call."[11]

Transferring the Eggs Back

The waiting for news of fertilization is nerve-wracking. About forty-eight hours after the egg harvest, the fertilized eggs, which must be kept at a constant temperature, are reinserted. "It's done in the hospital only because it's better for the patient to go to the eggs than for the eggs to go to the patient," says Jones.

The patient gets into position on an examining table. The doctor inserts a speculum to open up the vagina, checks the cervix, and wipes the cervix free of mucus to get a clear view of the entrance. He then announces over the intercom to the nurse in the laboratory that he is ready.

"Loading," she calls back, and fills a catheter with the patient's embryos and a little of the culture medium from the petri dish.

In the operating room, the doctor inserts the catheter deep into the uterus of the woman and pushes the plunger, shooting the embryos into inner space. The patient is then transferred to a stretcher and wheeled to the recovery room. The doctor is ready for the next hopeful patient.

"I guess some people think the way they do it at Norfolk is barbaric," says Caren. "They have you on your hands and knees with your rear end up in the air. They insert a needle into the uterus really fast and you lie down gently. They put everybody in the same room, and you stay there for about four hours."

When the baby factory empties out, the patients go back to their hotel to rest. The next day most of them go home, hoping they are pregnant.

But even at home the medical routine continues. To create a friendly environment for the embryo, the woman keeps taking progesterone shots, which were started a day or two after the laparoscopy and last for seven days. If she is lucky enough to get pregnant, progesterone shots are then continued weekly for eighteen weeks. For ten days after she gets home, the woman has to draw blood every other day. The blood is stored in the freezer until is it shipped by Federal Express to Norfolk. There the blood undergoes a pregnancy test via hormonal studies. The news of pregnancy or no pregnancy is conveyed by phone.

"You sit and wait," says Caren, "and about four o'clock the next day, you get that awful phone call: 'I'm sorry it is negative.' "

Caren gave up on *in vitro*, gave up on fertility pills, and had almost given up on ever having a baby when she got pregnant and had a "miracle" baby the old-fashioned way.

The Pain of Failure

Tim and Cindy Connors have been through the *in vitro* procedure three times at the Genetic and IVF Clinic in Fairfax, Virginia, but without any luck. At Fairfax, the egg retrieval is done without surgery. Instead, the ripe follicles are located by means of ultrasound, so the patient avoids both the general anesthesia and the hole in the abdomen. Guided to the ripe follicles by the pictures on the television screen, the physician penetrates the vaginal wall with a needle that sucks up the eggs. In Tim's opinion, the procedure was minor.

"It was very easy doing what we did," he says. "All you do is go in and lie down on the table and—"

Cindy interrupts him, a bit indignant. "It was easy for you. You just did it in a jar."

Even though Tim and Cindy used donor sperm for the IVF procedures because of Tim's "lousy" semen, he still gave a sample. Sometimes, if there is an abundance of eggs, the doctor will put the husband's deficient sperm with one or two of the eggs and of course, implant them if miraculously they fertilize. Tim is aware that the likelihood of that happening is minimal. "There is no way in hell—it is so low," he confesses. "But at the same time I can kid myself. I always give a specimen."

Even with ultrasound, IVF is not a piece of cake, but Tim and Cindy both agree that it was harder on the mind and emotions than on their bodies.

"We got very excited about it the first time," says Tim. "The second time we didn't, and it still hurt. The last time we did it was devastating. We have done it now three times, and we're taking the summer off. We just don't have the psychic energy. We tried to keep it in perspective, but still you wait for that phone call, and when you get the no, your heart just drops."

"Tim goes crazy," says Cindy. "And I would rather start my period than go back for the pregnancy test. They tell you they will call about five o'clock, but they call the people who have good news first. They don't tell you that, but we have all figured it out. You wait and wait for the phone to ring and they don't call, and all you can think about is that they are calling all the good people, saying 'Congratulations, it worked.' That part is very depressing."

It is difficult for everybody.

Dr. Robert Stillman has done his share of *in vitro* procedures at George Washington University Hospital and has had successes, but he has also faced many disappointments.

"We sometimes feel like we failed. We should be doing this better. But basically, if you've done as well as you can and haven't succeeded, maybe it is outside your capabilities. Nature, unfortunately in a way, still has an important role here."

When Susan and John Chambers decided to try external fertilization, Susan who had been through a lot already, approached it with cautious optimism. There was a reasonable chance it might help overcome her undefined problem, and it was almost certain to give John's sperm a better chance of fertilizing an egg.

Since the sperm are put right into the petri dish with the egg, the fertilizing cells do not have to swim very far. "You dump it right in there and any dummy can find the egg—even a blind pig will eventually find an acorn," Susan quips irreverantly.

Because Susan ovulated so well, the doctor decided to follow a slightly simpler procedure called an egg snatch. This is like *in vitro* except that the ovaries are stimulated with the less powerful Clomid instead of Pergonal, so fewer eggs are produced.

"We went in and had it done. I had a laparoscopy—it was my second or third; I ended up having six—and they got two eggs. Then they took John's sperm and I went home, recuperating."

John and Susan, each with his or her own fears and feelings, were sitting at home the Saturday morning after the egg retrieval when the hospital called with good news: The eggs had fertilized. Would they please come in and have the embryos implanted?

They were closer to a pregnancy than ever before. After six years of treatments, finally the beginning of life. It was fantastic, but, says Susan, "I felt awful. It sounds weird, but in a way it would have been nice to think the process was over. You want to get pregnant very badly, but in another way, you want an end to the kind of stress you feel you're under—the constant striving, striving, striving, another month, another procedure, another pill. Well, I thought, this will be it, I can put it to rest. But it wasn't; it opened up IVF. I felt, 'Oh damn!' I should have been happy, but there was an enormous sadness to it. It just meant I had to take a deep breath and keep going. So we schlepped to the hospital."

The embryos were transferred into Susan's womb, and another round of even worse waiting started.

Says Sarah Peters, who went through two unsuccessful attempts, "The wait is the most amazing experience in the world. You know that in some sense you're pregnant. There is life there. I walked in the park, talking to these little guys inside. You're waiting to see if they'll live. It is truly bizarre. While you're optimistic, it's very wonderful, and as soon as you feel your body change—and I could feel my body change—you could tell the pregnancy was no longer proceeding. It was like every month for the past five years, where it would be awful to get your period. But magnify it by a hundred. It wasn't exactly like a death, because you didn't know the person. But the letdown, and feeling your body die. . . ."

Because of Sarah's age her doctor refused to perform any more *in vitro* procedures on her. She and Steve are now trying for a surrogate baby.

Susan did not have any luck either. The embryos did not take. She got her period two weeks later.

"So there is that sadness too. You know you've come very, very close. That's as close as you can come to being pregnant, and when it doesn't work, it is not so good," Susan says with the understatement of an exhausted person.

Who are the people who after years and years of disappointments are still willing to take another dizzying ride on the emotional roller coaster? They have been studied by psychologists and described in abstract, scientific-sounding terms, but their attitude is best summed up by psychologist Susan Mikesell. Couples who will go to the nth degree to have a baby remind her, she says, of "people who deal with cancer, the fighters who decide they are not going to be consumed by the cancer. That's the reason they will go through some treatments that seem really outrageous and even masochistic. It isn't just the goal of having the baby. The biggest thing is wanting something and feeling that they not only have a right to, but they have something to offer: 'I really think I'll make a good parent.' "

L. D. Applegarth, who leads support groups for IVF couples in San Mateo, California, found that women in IVF programs frequently "view themselves as frustrated and driven." Not a surprising finding.

The Costs of IVF

But it takes more than drive to go through *in vitro* fertilization. It also takes money.

Each *in vitro* cycle costs about $5,000, and the money has to be paid up front. That is just the medical expense; it does not include transportation, time off from work, possible hotel accommodations, et cetera. Most couples have to go through more than one cycle. Seven is not unheard of.

Said Nan Tilton, the mother of *in vitro* twins, "We were lucky. We could afford it. One woman I heard about lived on hot dogs for a year to be able to pay for it. Another couple sold everything they had and came to Norfolk in a trailer. Other people mortgaged their homes."[12]

To some infertile couples, the money means little, even if they do not have much of it.

Mark Dooley, twenty-eight, who is in the motorcycle performance parts business, is married to Melinda, thirty-four, of San Bernardino County, California. She had one blocked tube and experienced the disappointment of a tubal pregnancy that destroyed the other and left her with no chance of conceiving naturally. "We thought back then that we wouldn't be able to have a baby at any price," said Mark. "People who can conceive naturally are bound to say, 'Gosh, five thousand dollars is a lot of money.' But for Melinda and me, five thousand dollars seems like nothing.''[13]

Health insurance companies, calling the *in vitro* procedure experimental, tend not to cover it. However, infertility support groups like Resolve are lobbying for a change, and already a few states, like Maryland, require insurance companies to pay for *in vitro* procedures. At Norfolk, Howard Jones observes that "insurance companies are doing better than they were before—seventy-five percent are getting health insurance coverage, but only twenty-five percent get full coverage and fifty percent get partial coverage." Even companies that do not officially provide coverage pay for more than they may realize. Many of the steps in the *in vitro* process are not specific to the procedure. Blood tests, sonograms, pelvic examinations, and so on are normally covered by insurance, and the *in vitro* physicians do not necessarily tell the insurer that these routine procedures have been performed in connection with an "experimental procedure."

In Vitro for Male Problems

When *in vitro* was first used as a therapy for infertility, only women with no fallopian tubes were candidates for IVF. Doctors wanted to demonstrate to the outside world that only they and not a lucky accident could have caused the pregnancy. Some physicians even insisted that the blocked tubes be removed surgically before *in vitro* attempts in order to leave no doubt as to how conception occurred. Soon, however, women who had defective tubes were allowed to participate, and now women with unexplained infertility, like Susan Chambers, can try *in vitro* as the last option.

While *in vitro* is used as a therapy to overcome more and more female problems of conception, it has also become a boon to men with minimal sperm. Because life is made easier for the sperm, which does not have to struggle through the female reproductive system, men who earlier had little chance of becoming biological fathers are given a lease on new life.

Says Dr. Chihal, "Most of the time IVF is to correct a female problem, but more and more it is for male infertility therapy. It gives us the ultimate functional test: Can this man's sperm fertilize this woman's egg? If they can, we have a realistic chance at fertility; if they can't, we have to change gears and go to donor insemination or suggest adoption."

"If a man has ten million motile sperm in the ejaculate, then they will attempt to do an IVF," says Dr. Lanasa. "What they have discovered is that a normal man, where the count is eighty million, one hundred million, two hundred million, or whatever, probably needs only twenty-five to fifty thousand sperm per egg. The quality of his sperm is better. But in a man who has a low count, his sperm is probably deficient, and it takes more sperm per egg to succeed. Initially [when trying *in vitro* for male problems] they were using the same number of sperm as for "normal" men, and they weren't getting success. They started to increase the number of sperm per egg and increased their success rate. But even then," he cautions, "you look at best at twenty percent pregnancy rates with IVF for male infertility."

In vitro fertilization has become an option for subfertile men, but it is still the woman who has to compensate for the man's deficiencies.

When Matt and Betty Peterson did not get pregnant, they discussed artificial insemination by donor but decided against it. The only other option was *in vitro*. They enrolled at the Genetic and IVF Clinic in Fairfax, Virginia, on an outpatient basis, and then the hormone shots started, one every evening around six o'clock. Matt became an expert at loading the syringe and giving Betty a shot in the buttock, but sticking to the schedule for the injections was not so easy.

"We had to do it in some very strange places," Matt recounts, laughing. "Once, after hiking in the Shenandoah, we stopped at a truck stop, and right there in the car between the truckers, we put a coat over Betty and watched the people coming by as we were loading the hormones in the dark.

"It was a real busy stop. This guy parked right next to us, and he didn't get out of his car, so we had to sit there and wait. He was probably thinking we were having oral sex or something. Finally, he got out and went to the bathroom. Then it didn't take much, just poke it in there."

Betty could never "just poke it in there" herself, although she tried when Matt couldn't get home from work on time.

When sonography was needed to check on the size of the ovaries, Betty would get up early in the morning and, with her bladder full and her bowel empty, repair to the hospital.

Finally after about ten days of shots, blood tests, and sonograms and urine analysis, it was time for the egg retrieval. Betty had two ripe eggs, but Matt's sperm failed to fertilize them. That was supposed to be the end, but because their insurance had picked up more of the cost than expected, they decided to do it one more time—more shots, more early mornings, more sonograms, two eggs retrieved and mixed with sperm of doubtful ability.

To divert themselves while waiting for the news of fertilization or no fertilization after the second attempt, Matt and Betty went to watch a golf tournament. Betty called the clinic from the tenth green.

"There were several people waiting to use the phone," Matt remembers. "She was put on hold and then they finally came back and, lo and behold, the eggs had fertilized. We could have run out and kissed the golfers. We couldn't believe it.

"It was a tremendous thing. It took a lot of pressure off me: There is a chance, there is a possibility."

The embryos were implanted but did not "stick."

"Once the eggs fertilized, it was nobody's fault, absolutely nobody's fault. It was just nature not allowing the transfer to take. Once we got into *in vitro*, it was no longer his problem," Betty says loyally.

Matt and Betty were, in spite of not having achieved a pregnancy, elated that Matt's sperm was capable of fertilizing Betty's eggs; and when their gynecologist said, "If I were you, I would take out every loan—just go for it, spend twenty thousand dollars on it," they decided to try again.

"The first time, it was going to be once only," Betty confesses, "Then it was twice and we got the fertilized egg, and it was like, whoa, we've got to go again. It was like rolling the dice, it really was."

"Every time we went to the clinic, we would hold hands as we drove down there," says Matt, "And on the way we would tell God, 'If you give us a child, we'll raise it in your ways.' "

The deal with God did not work out. Once again Betty did not get pregnant. But their attitude was "why quit now?" They did it again. Four eggs were harvested; they were all fertilized and all put back in Betty's womb. Matt *knew* it was going to work this time.

"Do you want to hear why?" he asks, not quite sure he wants to tell. "Well, it is farfetched, but I really believe this. I have a cousin in Minnesota who is a more devout Methodist than I am, and I shared this with him. He told me, 'My wife has a prayer list, and when we put things on there, those prayers are answered.' When he said that, I knew it was going to work, I really knew it was going to work. There is no scientific evidence that after all our failures . . . but there was in the corner of my heart an inner peace that this time it's going to work. I continued my prayers, and I know they did, too.''

Betty got pregnant, with twins no less.

"I was very surprised when we got the good news,'' says Matt, "but I also wasn't surprised, because I thought, 'God did come through.' '' It was not exactly by immaculate conception.

"Ten days after the transfer, you go back for a blood test,'' Betty explains, "then again two days later, then two more days and two more days, so you have blood tests all the time. Then after you get pregnant, you take injections for three months—LH first, and then you switch to progesterone.''

"Betty has needle marks all over her body from two hundred to three hundred injections,'' Matt reveals, and he is not even counting the hundreds of times she has been pricked for blood tests.

But Betty agrees with her husband: "I definitely think it was God's work here. I do remember, though, after the first times, crying and crying—Why would God do this to us? There was a lot of crying over failures, and at times it seems so all-consuming. You get so wrapped up in it, but when we became pregnant, I quickly forgot the year and the problems there.''

Betty gives little thought to the fact that she went through all the trying procedures not because she had a problem, but because Matt did. She is thrilled. She has Matt take pictures of her stomach in front of the mirror "to get the double effect or something.'' Matt laughs. "She is as happy as can be.''

Religion and Infertility

Susan Chambers was tired and disappointed after the unsuccessful egg snatch, but not defeated. She and her doctor decided to try a full *in vitro* with Pergonal and hospital stay.

Susan responded abundantly to the Pergonal. She produced six eggs, "all beautiful eggs,'' and they all fertilized and were all put back in her uterus. After the transfer, she had to stay on her stomach for six hours, but did eight for safety's sake.

"You don't know if you can move; you're trying so hard to make them stick that you don't want to sneeze.''

When she got home, she took no chances. She stayed in bed as much as possible.

Susan claims she had no expectations about the *in vitro* attempt and was just "trying to have my head screwed on straight." She had already been through so much and had been trying to reach some kind of acceptance of her predicament.

"I'm a Catholic," she says, "not a strong Catholic, but I carry it with me. Over the years I have prayed in various ways. I started out praying I would get pregnant, then praying that whatever my fate was to more or less make it happen and make me able to accept it. I said this long novena, a novena to Mary. I said it to Mary because I thought, being a mother she would understand—this sounds kind of weird—what it would mean to me to be a mother." Susan laughs at herself. "So it was a fifty-four-day novena—twenty-seven days of petition and twenty-seven days of thanksgiving. I did all that and nothing happened. At one point I was really anxious. If this is not going to work, just give me some understanding and then I will return to some kind of state of serenity or peace within myself. Well, that didn't happen either."

Religion can both help and aggravate the problems of infertility. People who are strongly religious will often see infertility as punishment for their sins.

Tim and Cindy Connors are also Catholics, and Tim's mind did "stupid things" when he learned about his infertility. "My Catholicism taught me I must have done something very wrong, and in my mind the guilt was coming on and all sorts of hard feelings came along with that."

Some people lose their faith.

Said one woman, "I always had faith that my belief in God would help me through anything. I always thought that if you prayed hard enough for something, you would get it. But when you wholeheartedly go to church every day and then find out that your tubes are blocked just after tuboplasty, it is real easy to become an atheist.[14]

The Catholic Church is officially opposed to all "unnatural" forms of conception, which include *in vitro*. And that adds an extra strain on the faithful who choose to ignore the rules.

Says Cindy, "I felt that suddenly the church didn't want me because we did something they were saying was wrong. The one thing we were always taught, to have children, was the one thing we couldn't achieve, and now we're being told that, in an effort to achieve it, we are doing something wrong. It hits you hard."

Says Tom, "God's plans are going to come to fruition regardless of what we do. We are just trying to do everything *we* can to achieve something we want very badly and what the church has always taught us to want very badly."

On the Edge and to the Limit of Science

After the embryo transfer, Susan went back to work—carefully.

"I was so good. One flight of stairs, and I would take the elevator. I wouldn't carry my briefcase. John came up to get my briefcase every night. You figure you'll just sit here and not move, you won't breathe too hard, just stay and let the thing stick. You're really intense about this. It was incredible, it was crazy, but it means enough to you to do that."

In spite of her extreme precautions, she started to spot and thought her period was coming, but the hospital wanted her to come in for a blood test.

She had a positive pregnancy reading, the first one ever. She had blood tests for a few days to check on the hormone levels, which are supposed to rise steeply with pregnancy, but in Susan's case they did not. Susan had been right, she got her period.

"I was rather blown away when it didn't work. You always wonder what you did that screwed it up. You think, 'I played Ring Around the Rosie with my nieces. Damn it, I shouldn't have done that,' or that one day I carried my own briefcase—'It was too heavy; I shouldn't have done that.' You know it's stupid. Women get pregnant, they dig ditches, they pick cotton, and that does not screw up their implantation. It was absurd."

The *in vitro* procedure works like clockwork these days except for one aspect, the implantation. Nobody is sure what the difficulty is there. Dr. Chihal thinks "that part of the problem with IVF is the condition of the uterine lining at the time of the embryo transfer. The woman, of course, receives a large number of medications—in our case commonly clomiphene and Pergonal, so she has abnormally high estrogen levels and abnormal progesterone levels, and it is entirely possible that we are making the uterine lining a more hostile environment for the embryo than in a natural cycle. But all this is strictly hypothetical."

Another major disappointment for Susan and John: six beautifully fertilized eggs implanted, a positive pregnancy reading, and not one of the embryos developed.

"If one has tried *in vitro* and it is not successful," says Constance Shapiro, "there is a feeling of real death that has occurred, a feeling of barrenness that is worse than before, a feeling of the inability of one's body to nurture that is, I think, horrible for women who want more than anything to nurture. I think it is dramatically different from the usual agonies of infertility."

Even John, who describes himself as an optimist, was dejected.

"First the procedure takes so long, and you have to do so many things to be ready for it. When they fertilize an egg and put it back in the body, for the first time you know an egg has been fertilized—you never knew that before—and that in your mind brings you closer than ever before. Then you go one step further, and the reading indicates that there is a pregnancy, and then to lose that! It's like losing a child."

Susan had neither become pregnant nor found serenity, so when her doctor told her that a Dr. John Parsons was coming over from England to do what was then an experimental procedure, harvesting eggs using only sonographic ultrasound and no laparoscopy, Susan volunteered to be the subject of the experiment.

"Coming from a medical family, just being inquisitive about medical things, as I went through infertility, part of it I found fascinating . . . and in a way, going through *in vitro*, I felt we were on the edge of medical science. It was extremely interesting."

For Susan, her third attempt at fertilization outside the body became a scientific as well as religious test.

"I had it all mixed up with religion," says Susan. "I had had the feeling for a while that God had turned away from me, that he wasn't listening to me, and that made me feel lonely and isolated. So I asked him to turn back to me and to show me that he had turned back to me."

For the experiment to work, Susan's menstrual cycle had to be coordinated with Dr. Parsons' arrival in December 1985. So first she went on birth control to stop ovulation, and then megadoses of Pergonal to get ovulation going again at the desired time. It was a close call, but it worked.

Susan and John went to the hospital. John gave his sperm sample and got into his surgical gown, and Susan was sedated with Demerol but stayed awake during the procedure.

"Of course, with a new procedure there were dozens of people in there—the radiologist, all the nurses, all these fellows, and three doctors," says Susan. "With all these people in the room, you can't be a shrinking violet. Here you are exposed to the world; in a way you feel part of the machinery, kind of detached, kind of impersonal. I mean, you're trying to maintain some sense of your personness, and then there are all those people looking at you in an experimental way.''

John was right there with Susan and could observe what was happening on the TV monitor. Susan wanted to look, too, but she was too groggy from the Demerol.

Dr. Parsons located an egg and, says Susan, "They got so excited—'Look there's one!' And there you are with a machine round your stomach, and they are really into it; you're kind of an afterthought—'Oh, oh, are you okay?' '' She laughs. "You want to say, 'Whoa, guys, there is a person down here.' Sometimes they tend to lose track of that. The patient is almost dehumanized.''

John found the procedure "interesting and fascinating." "You sit there sort of transfixed. You don't even pay attention to Susan—you're watching the screen.''

The experiment was a success. Dr. Parsons retrieved three eggs, and they all fertilized and were implanted.

A step forward for medical science perhaps, but no pregnancy. The embryos did not attach themselves to the uterine wall, and Susan got her period.

Neither science nor God came through for Susan that time, but she did not lose her faith. "I don't think I ever left God, although he may have felt that way. I tried to reassure him,'' she says and bursts into laughter.

But Susan did decide to give up on science. She sat down and wrote her doctor a thirteen-page dear-John letter, "telling him I was cutting him loose. I thought we should bag it at that point.''

Susan had become friendly with her doctor over the years, and she and John occasionally saw him socially, so she delivered the letter to him personally but asked him not to read it in her presence. He did though, and slowly went through their history of relationship. When he finished, he got up from his chair and stared silently out the window.

"I thought he would say, 'This is it; there is nothing I can do with you,' '' Susan says.

Instead the doctor said, "What do you want me to do? How can I help you through this?'' That was only the prelude to a new suggestion.

Susan's fertility problems had never been pinpointed—she ovulated well, her tubes were not blocked, her slight endometriosis had been cleared up, so there was no reason why she could not conceive. John's problem, however, was clear. His sperm was marginal. Assuming that Susan's body functioned normally and that she was able to conceive with viable sperm, the doctor wanted her to try artificial insemination by donor. "I know it is an emotionally tense time, but it is only going to be six months. I think you should at least try it," he advised.

"I had been trying for eight and a half years, so I was really tired, and there is always so much emotional intensity you have to put forth. But I thought, 'Maybe you're right, maybe I owe it to myself.' So I said, 'Okay, I'll do it.' "

But that was not all. Before he started the inseminations, he wanted to do a diagnostic laparoscopy to make sure her insides were in perfect order.

"You're telling me I'm going to have surgery!" Susan shot back at the doctor. "I'm just getting over the fact that I didn't get pregnant after the last IVF, and you're telling me you want to do diagnostic laparoscopy?"

A week later Susan was on the operating table.

She knew she was close to ovulation, and while her physician was looking around inside her, he found a mature egg, which he snatched. Again John's sperm fertilized the egg, but again the embryo did not take.

Then it was time for artificial insemination—six months of it and no pregnancy. And that was really it.

"I'm a fairly strong person, although you reach the point sometimes where you feel you're letting yourself down, your body is not working. I felt perhaps I was letting John down, and then there was my doctor. He really wanted me to get pregnant and I knew that, and he had his professional pride, and I thought maybe I'm disappointing him by stopping."

But Susan was also disappointed with herself. "If I could have willed my body into working, I would have done it. I think the desire for a woman to have a child is incredible. It is intellectual and emotional, but the disappointment you feel when you can't have children is not only intellectual and emotional, it's physiological. Your body is saying every single month that you can have a child, but you're not having a child and it is very difficult to deal with. I wanted to have a child. I wanted to carry my own children. That was the driving force behind me. I wanted to hold my children close to me."

Susan has a child, a beautiful little boy that she loves dearly. He is adopted. Still . . .

"I can hold Riley and I can love Riley, but sometimes this sadness comes over me when I look at him. "I couldn't hold you as close as I want to hold you. I couldn't eat carrots to make your eyes pretty. I couldn't drink milk . . ." Tears well up in Susan's eyes and her voice breaks. "There is nothing I can ever . . . I can't have that with you."

Susan is sorry that she did not manage to give birth to her child, but she does not regret having explored every option open to the infertile. She is still friendly with her doctor. She had him over for a barbecue dinner when it was all over, and by chance it became the night when she purged her life of the infertility nightmare. She was preparing a rack of lamb on the grill but could not get the charcoal started. "I was looking around for something to get the charcoal started," Susan says, "and I thought "Aha, I've got all those temperature charts—years and years worth. And I put them under the charcoal."

But there was one thing Susan did not burn. "In one of my *in vitros* I had them take a picture of the fertilized eggs. I always thought it was the closest thing to having my own child that I would ever see, and I'm right."

Still, Susan and John have not completely ruled out trying to have a baby again when science has something new to offer, and science is working on it.

5

Science Creates a New Business

THEY ARE DRESSED IN BLUE SCRUB GARB, GATHERED AT THE AP-
pointed hour—6:00 A.M. at the hospital. Their ritual is called
gamete intrafallopian transfer, a name whose acronym, GIFT,
makes it seem less scientific and more miraculous. Still, it costs
$4,000. The object of their combined attention, the barren woman.
She and her husband have already mastered the seven analysis,
hysterosalpinogram (to see if her tubes are blocked), the fertility
drugs (Clomid and Pergonal) and the sonograms. These are the
steps by which the scientists seize control of what used to be the
woman's personal menstrual cycle.

"Here at Georgetown," the doctor explains, "the shot of Pergonal
is given by the husband at home. I've found it's very successful.
Sometimes the male feels left out; this allows him to play a role, to
provide important psychological support."

Timing is everything when you are trying both to control and
mimic Mother Nature. The husband's sperm has been washed and
carefully prepared in the lab next door.

Today the woman has reached the crucial step, gamete retrieval,
which will decide if she has pleased the gods and science enough

for them to make her pregnant. She has learned to say "laparoscopy" without hesitation, and she is told that she is full of good mature eggs.

"In one woman the ovaries blew up as big as a football. But that was just one woman. The problem is we're trying to override Mother Nature," says Dr. DiMattina about the hyperstimulation of the ovaries. "She wants only one egg and we want several so that it will result in a clinical pregnancy, [but] multiple pregnancies are a risk. The female body was not made to have litters. With all the procedures that is a risk . . . We have to find the right recipe."

The egg hunt begins with the physician cutting a tiny hole in the woman's abdomen. Sliding the laparoscope through the abdomen and into her ovaries, he checks for a blister-like follicle. With the spears of his trade protruding from her stomach like giant knitting needles from a ball of yarn, he pokes and finds one.

"I'm the only one in the country who has this special needle," DiMattina boasts, clearly enjoying his first-on-the-block superiority. "Here at Georgetown, the entire procedure is done through this needle. . . . I trained at Kings College with Dr. John Parsons. We call it a JP needle."

He pushes his one-of-a-kind needle through the follicle wall— "Can you see it collapse?" he asks. Quickly the eggs are sucked out, harvested through the catheter.

It's a fairly bloodless procedure. The eggs are transferred to a tiny glass petri dish, hand labeled "eggs," and passed to the embryologist, who, via a high-powered microscope, attests to their vitality. Eight eggs in all. Four are rated "5"—good maturity— and the others are not so good. They are all placed on a warming plate at the temperature of the human body; they will sit there for no more than twenty minutes.

The laparoscope still protrudes from the woman's abdomen while an assistant retrieves her husband's sperm, which will travel into her body via another catheter. The sperm and eggs will both go directly to her fallopian tubes—two eggs in one tube, two eggs in the other. Actual fertilization takes place in the woman's body, making GIFT more acceptable to some religious groups.

The doctor positions the catheter and fires out the command "Inject."

"The catheter is really beautiful," he says. "Once she's got those eggs in the catheter, you can count one minute and I'll guarantee I'll get those eggs in there. I don't know why others can't do that."

The doctor's success rate so far with GIFT is one full-term pregnancy out of eight tries, but he is hopeful, competitive, and smart about what he repeatedly calls a "crap shoot."

"The bottom line is, what's the pregnancy rate? The gold standard in this country is Norfolk. But IVF is not very successful. One-third of the women who have gone through IVF have never had a clinical pregnancy. We're much above the national average for egg collection. The average is 3.4 eggs per patient; we're around five."

With brains and technology behind him, DiMattina is confident.

"With this new vaginal probe, I'm excited as hell; it's almost like sticking your head in the pelvis and looking around. It's gorgeous!

"This is what separates my program—these consultants to George-town. Dr. John Parsons predicted that men would have babies and the phone rang off the wall—transvestites, everyone called here to offer their bodies as the first."

DiMattina is frustrated that he has to keep such a low profile on his work at a Catholic university.

" '20/20' was supposed to be here, but at the last minute the university decided against it," he says. "They are afraid someone might find it offensive. I'm a Catholic—well, not the best Catholic—and I don't see anything wrong with it. I'm not handling human life; I'm handling the ingredients of human life. This is straight—no hocus-pocus."

Dr. DiMattina, who loves his job—"There's so much you can do, go anywhere you want, go out on a limb as far as you want"—is hawking his skills at a public lecture accompanied by a film illustrating GIFT, one of the newest fertility rituals. Competition among fertility experts is heating up.

Entreprenuerial IVF

Infertility clinics are being created all over the United States. It takes only a business card in addition to the M.D. to qualify as an infertility specialist.

"How many gynecologists have obstetrics, gynecology, and infertility on their cards?" Dr. Robert Stillman of George Washington University Hospital ponders. "They don't put down 'paraneonatology, high risk obstetrics.' They put 'infertility.' Why? Because it is hard to make things worse in infertility. The patient doesn't get not pregnant. She is already not pregnant."

Matt and Betty Peterson's gynecologist had "fertility" on his card, but, says Betty, "I don't think he was a fertility specialist as such. He was good at referring us, but we would often tell him what was going on at the *in vitro* center. I'm not putting him down at all, but I don't think he really knows."

Just as follicles respond to Pergonal, entrepreneurs respond to money. IVF clinics are proliferating. There are about 200 worldwide, and more are on the way. The American Fertility Society keeps tabs on those in the United States but does not regulate them or rate their success. It does contend that of the 9,500 self-identified reproductive specialists worldwide a "substantial number" have not produced a single live birth.

Of the seventy-five IVF clinics in the United States, about sixty-five are at university centers. The rest have been established by investors or are associated with already existing commercial hospitals. The fertility industry is a $400 to $500 million a year business, and the amount is bound to increase as infertility rates rise due to venereal disease, pollution, occupational hazards, and delayed childbirth.

IVF clinics are not required to meet any specific medical qualifications before opening their doors, and some clinics have nothing to recommend them.

"There are some entrepreneurs that are bogus," says Stillman. "They make money like some people selling swampland in Florida. That's an unfortunate spin-off of every profession and every technology, and there are certainly people doing that."

The most successful program in the world is IVF Australia.

"It is a group from Australia that comes to the United States and sets up units here," explains Dr. Mark Geier of Genetics Consultants, who made a few unsuccessful *in vitro* attempts before he gave up. "The Australian technology is the best in the world. The general approach is the same, but the details are better. They seem to have a higher success rate, and they have the largest program in the world. They have had three or four thousand pregnancies. Australia did the first frozen embryo birth; they are really in the forefront of what's going on."

So far, IVF Australia has set up clinics in Port Chester, New York, and in Birmingham, Alabama, and Dr. Geier is in negotiations to open another. IVF Australia successfully floated stock to start the clinics, but because the cost of equipment is high and it also costs a lot to train personnel and operate the clinics, they have yet to see a profit. A lot of customers are required if investors' seed money is not to drain away in a stillborn enterprise.

"We invest heavily in public relations," says Vicki Baldwin, founder of IVF Australia in this country, who herself had a test tube baby while living in Australia. She uses standard PR techniques like direct mailings, seminars, and flyers to attract the attention of gynecologists who will refer their patients to the clinics.[1]

Other hospitals are following suit. Mt. Sinai Hospital in New York City held an IVF seminar that attracted 270 potential customers, corresponding to potential fees of over $1 million.

IVF Australia obviously relies on a good and tested procedure, with a 50 percent chance of pregnancy after four *in vitro* treatments, but the procedure is not everything.

"These procedures happen to be operator sensitive," Charles Hartman of CW Group, a New York venture capital firm that specializes in medical technologies, told the *New York Times*. "It is like a famous neurosurgeon who is able to do a procedure that his best students cannot do very well."[2]

Dr. Geoffrey Sher of the Northern Nevada Family Fertility Clinic agrees: "The best IVF doctors are like master chefs. Very subtle differences in the recipe can make the difference between success and failure."[3]

Many new IVF clinics are fly-by-night operations, according to Stillman, who is associated with George Washington University Hospital, a teaching hospital. "There are some entrepreneurial groups—physicians and backers of physicians—who have tried to take *in vitro* fertilization into the marketplace, and they have done extremely poorly for the most part, in large part because they don't have any comprehension or understanding of the effort, the financial cost, and the background."

Whether or not the clinics are successful, they are all searching for bodies to make babies and money on. Says Dr. Sher, "The whole thing in IVF is numbers. You need to go above a certain threshold to make a lot of money."[4] With over 150 clinics out there looking for the big numbers, it is a buyer beware situation.

The best advertising is, of course, a high success rate, but those clinics starting up have no figures to quote and may therefore cite the best figures around, which is only unethical if they do not point out that they are quoting somebody else's track record. "Beware of centers that say their expected birth rate will be twenty-five percent," says Dr. Richard Marrs of Cedars Sinai Hospital in Los Angeles. "Their expected birth rate is zero until they have produced a baby."[5]

"The couple should demand to know the take-home baby rate," advises Lori B. Andrews of the American Bar Foundation.[6]

Some clinics are leery about giving out information about themselves. According to Dr. Bellina, a random check of thirty *in vitro* clinics revealed that less than half freely provided information on request to the callers.[7] Some clinics insist on seeing the patient's medical records first, which means that the patient is already halfway in the bag before she has any idea of what she can expect.

There is good reason to be skeptical of promises from almost any clinic because, according to Dr. Sher, only three clinics nationwide are responsible for 50 percent of the IVF babies born in the United States.[8] That does not necessarily mean that a small clinic like Dr. Chihal's in Dallas, which will see no more than two IVF patients a day, has less success. In fact, a patient may get more personalized care than in high-volume centers like Norfolk with a number of rotating doctors and series of patients. But knowing whether a particular center is reputable or has a credible record of success is difficult.

"If I were in a couple's shoes," says Dr. John Fletcher, bioethicist at the National Institutes of Health, "I would get a trusted consultant to guide me in selecting fertility services."[9]

The Push to Produce

Many of the established clinics have long waiting lists and are not looking for additional customers. However, listening to the stories of the infertile, it is hard not to suspect that fertility specialists often push their patients into procedures that they may not be thrilled about.

"I have had couples tell me they get to a point where they are ready to stop, where they can live with childlessness, only to be pushed by physicians to keep trying," says Lori B. Andrews.[10]

Susan Chambers, who went through nine years of what seems like medical and psychological torture, appears to be a case in point.

"I came to a point where I was worried what it was going to do to Susan," says her husband. "I got to the point where I didn't care whether we stopped or not." But Susan pressed on.

When it was all over, "I was so emotionally tired," she says. "I had never before felt as tired in my life, a kind of permeating emotional tiredness which is really difficult to deal with. You feel some of that throughout, but at the very end, that's when I started to feel really, really tired, like I was running on an empty tank or the fumes. I had no strength to go on.''

And yet she never felt pushed into anything by her doctor.

"Maybe if you put yourself into the hands of the doctor and let him control your medical destiny, maybe it can happen, but what kind of thinking person would do that? Maybe some do; I could never do that. I had to feel that I was the one who controlled it. I was the one who said, 'I will do IVF; I'll do this and I'll stop.' ''

But for romance writer Kitty Sidler and many others, it is a no-questions-asked situation. "Our position was very clear," she says. "We do everything available. I never question the wisdom of doing a procedure.''

Infertile people are notoriously vulnerable and desperately want to believe that they can be helped. Says Dr. Joseph Lanasa, "Some patients want you to do 'everything possible,' so therefore they let themselves have things done to them that are of questionable value. One of the hardest things to tell patients is that you do *not* have an alternative for them. There are patients out there grasping for straws, for that pot of gold at the end of the rainbow, and they will let you put their head on backwards if they think it is going to give them a pregnancy.''

A couple that desperate to have a baby is easily persuaded that almost any risk is outweighed by the benefits. And they may not realize fully that what the doctor from his clinical perspective sees as reasonable may have consequences that are not discussed in medical textbooks.

Says feminist writer Julie Melrose, "There is a difference between the way the doctor defines a surgical procedure and the way a person experiences it. Doctors have a tendency to look at surgical procedures in a technical and mechanical way. If they see a way to manipulate the body to accomplish what they want without posing an extremely high risk, they define that procedure as a piece of cake. From their position as mechanics, it *is* a piece of cake, an easy procedure for them to perform.

"My feeling is that the human body has an integrity of its own and that it cannot be violated, even in a way that the doctor may see as minor, without there being physical and emotional consequences for the person on whom the surgery is performed.''[11]

It is standard practice in many IVF programs to have a psychologist on board to alert and prepare the patients for the ordeal and likely disappointment of external fertilization. Susan Mikesell, who is associated with the Columbia Hospital for Women in

Washington, D.C., has occasional moments of doubts when she counsels patients. "Sometimes I wonder about all this technology. Are we really doing people a big favor by having all this technology available to them? Yes, sometimes I do wonder what the heck we're doing, and why we don't tell people, 'That's enough!' "

"It is always the patient's choice," says Dr. Levitt. "It is their money, it is their choice, it is their option, and you have to give them all the options so they can understand and make the decision. The doctor should not be making the decision. I never say die, because I don't believe in that word, but I don't push them either. I won't say no, I won't say quit. If a person wants to keep going and you say stop, what are they going to do? Go to another doctor. You are not going to change their minds."

With minor variations that is what all doctors say: It is the patient's choice. Since infertile women wanting children are as ferocious in their desire to have children as lionesses guarding their cubs, it almost always means "What's next?"

Says Dr. Stillman, "Couples are vastly interested in using new technologies that can help where they haven't been helped before, and they are part of the problem. Often they will be pushing the physician, pushing the technologies that really may not be appropriate, and often they will not hear when the physician says, 'I think there are other things we should be doing before this.' There is a pressure among many people to say, 'I haven't tried everything if I haven't tried *in vitro.*' "

For the doctor "there are multiple pressures involved," Dr. Stillman points out. "Ego competition, to be first in an area, marketplace competition, patient pressures, the media and Resolve, and so on—all of those mixed into a very emotional and very trying time for the couple. Most physicians are cognizant of those pressures and try to minimize them, try to put the patients into appropriate procedures and into safe and effective modalities," he explains, lapsing into doctor-speak.

Physicians are naturally tempted to keep trying. Their reputations rest on their success, and achieving success is a great "high" to fertility specialists.

"When an infertility patient gets pregnant, that makes me ecstatic," says Dr. Jeffrey Levitt.

"I have found it to be very challenging, very rewarding when I see individuals who are infertile achieve the most important thing they want in life. It's a great feeling to see them get pregnant, using whatever technique is necessary. I get quite a lot of personal satisfaction out of doing this," says Dr. DiMattina.

And the patients who do get pregnant are immensely grateful.

Betty and Mark Peterson have great admiration for the doctors and staff at The Genetic and IVF Institute in Fairfax that gave them twins. "Those people are devoted—long hours, never a day off. It's incredible. They are there at seven-thirty in the morning and they would still be calling us at nine-thirty at night. They always had a cheerful face, never complained, and never had a negative attitude. When they saw those twins on the sonogram, and saw us crying and jumping up and down for joy, they told us, 'This is why we do it, these moments.' This is what keeps them going."

Patients occasionally begin to see the doctor who may make their wishes come true as godlike.

"Obviously," says David Glass, "when a doctor or a team of doctors is able to help a couple have a child, there is tremendous affection, gratitude, and respect."

But the doctors do not always succeed, and then . . .

"A lot of anger is directed at the doctor," Glass continues. "It's funny, every time you have several infertile couples getting together and talking about the situation, the caustic humor at the doctors' expense is really very amusing and pronounced and, the doctors would say, quite excessive and quite unfair. It is the combination of needing the doctor so much and wanting him to be godlike, to create miracles, and yet knowing that doctors can't and resenting them when they aren't."

"It is a wonderful, exciting, and fabulous job," says Dr. Stillman, "but in many ways it is a technical job. You have to go in, be careful, compulsive, make sure, support, get the job done. If it works, fabulous. If it doesn't, we have to do better. We are probably better off looking at ourselves as trained technicians and mechanics rather than as gods."

The infertility business is "a hard profession to be in," says psychologist Susan Mikesell, "because you have to deal with so many disappointments. For as many people as you get pregnant, you still have to deal with the people that you can't help. You have to deal with patients you have had for six or seven years. You just know there is nothing you can do. Doctors aren't well trained to deal with that kind of helplessness."

"It's very disappointing, but you have to keep going" is Dr. Stillman's response to failures.

Keep going seem to be the operative words in most infertility treatments, where neither the doctor nor the patient seems to know the word *stop*.

"Unfortunately, there are some physicians who are not as scrupulous and let themselves get swayed, and they will do things of questionable benefit to the patient," admits Dr. Lanasa. "It is the physician's personal decision, and that's part of the art of medicine; it's not purely science. I think that a lot of procedures—not just in infertility, but in anything in medicine—get abused by overuse."

"There have been abuses as far as *in vitro* fertilization is concerned," admits Dr. Pierre Asmar, in private practice in Annandale, Virginia. "For example, I'm not very impressed with the pregnancy rate for the use of *in vitro* fertilization for unexplained infertility. I think we have to stick to basics and limit ourselves to specific indications, and those indications have to be based on clinical studies to show us which situation would be the best. We shouldn't be carried away too far." And there's the rub. What is too far?

"The situation in human reproduction and the ethics of applying these new technologies in our society today are profoundly confused," says Dr. John Fletcher, bio-ethicist at the National Institutes of Health. "If you look in the literature, you find a lot of contending positions, but you don't find many people asking questions like: What is the prevailing morality and where are we going to end up? The dominant morality in the U.S. as far as these technologies are concerned is that the customer's ethics prevail."

In other words, if the patient or the patient's bank account does not say stop, a woman can chase babies until she is postmenopausal.

Frozen Embryos

Over the last decade there have been so many firsts in human reproduction that it is hard to keep track of them all. What was experimental a year or two ago is now routine procedure. One major advance has been the freezing of embryos.

More than two dozen babies had already been born from frozen embryos in Australia, Britain, the Netherlands, Israel, and West Germany when a boy who had started out life frozen in liquid nitrogen was born in Los Angeles on June 4, 1986, to Gary, a forty-seven-year-old physician, and his wife Monique, thirty-six.

Monique had had damaged fallopian tubes since the age of twenty-one and had tried *in vitro* three times unsuccessfully, when her doctor, Richard Marrs, then of Good Samaritan Hospital in Los Angeles, suggested they freeze four embryos that had been left over from the last procedure. Monique was skeptical but went along with Dr. Marrs' idea. She said, "I didn't want to grow to be eighty years old and childless and think there was something I could have done and didn't do."

Dr. Marrs put Monique's four embryos in a small refrigerator-like device controlled by a computer. The temperature was lowered by .03 degrees centigrade per minute until it reached −76 degrees. The embryos were then stored in liquid nitrogen at −196 degrees. When Monique ovulated later, the embryos were thawed and implanted in her uterus.

The baby boy that Monique gave birth to nine months later was "a healthy baby, normal in every way."[13]

Although the Catholic Church and a number of other groups are against embryo freezing (along with all other technology-assisted forms of conception) because the embryo's life is endangered, the technique has advantages. It is cheaper, and it simplifies the medical procedures necessary to create a pregnancy and is therefore less physically stressful for the potential mother.

The Embryo: Healthy or Harmed?

There is always the worry that the embryo will suffer damage when manipulated outside the body and result in a defective child. Cries of caution from ethicists and scientists were heard when IVF first became possible. At a symposium held in Washington, D.C., in 1971, James Watson, the Nobel Prize winner and discoverer of the double helix structure of DNA, warned Dr. Robert Edwards, "You can only go ahead with your work if you accept the necessity of infanticide. There are going to be a lot of mistakes. What are you going to do with the mistakes?" And ethicist Leon Kass argued, "It doesn't matter how many times the [test tube] baby is tested while in the mother's womb; they will never be certain the baby won't be born without a defect."[14]

Kass is right. There is no way to be sure that the test tube baby will be normal, but there are no guarantees of perfection in normal conception either. It appears that *in vitro* babies—even those from frozen embryos—do not differ from the normally conceived population. Dr. Frederick Wirth of the Eastern Virginia Medical School in Norfolk has conducted follow-up studies on 180 Norfolk *in vitro* babies. "We took *in vitro* patients and matched them with controls, looking at general risk factors for congenital malformations, and found that they were equally present in both infant populations."

The results of Dr. Wirth's study—the only carefully controlled such research in the world—are encouraging. Says Wirth, "We actually expected to find an increased coincidence of congenital malformation in babies conceived *in vitro*. We didn't find any difference at all. Unfortunately, we can't say with complete confidence, but we can say with a great deal of confidence that there is no difference."

Dr. Alan DeCherney of the Yale School of Medicine studied about fifty *in vitro* babies and came to the same tentative conclusion. "This is a short-term study about the outcome of their birth and a little bit into their lives—maybe six months—and they are no different from anyone else."

"Well, it is remarkable," says Dr. Wirth. "For centuries, for all of evolution in primates and in the lower animals we have evolved from, conception was done in a very protective environment—lower oxygen concentrations, no presence of light, very carefully controlled temperatures. And they take these gametes out and fertilize them at room temperature, and Howard Jones takes a picture with a flash of the fertilized eggs, and lo and behold . . . Absolutely incredible, if you think about it. To me it just verifies the strength of our genetic process and reproductive system. Absolutely incredible."

A larger and older *in vitro* population is needed for complete assurance of the safety of external fertilization. Since the oldest *in vitro* child in the world, Louise Brown, is only nine years old, nobody can tell if the mode of their conception will have negative consequences later in life. Even if the children are medically sound, it is not inconceivable that psychological problems stemming from the fact that they are "different," having been conceived by extraordinary means, will show up when the children go to school.

"At least from my perspective," says Nan Tilton, whose *in vitro* twins, Todd and Heather, are four years old and in nursery school, "it seems that they will only feel as different as they are made to feel. But there will obviously be some things that come up at points in their lives, especially during adolescence."

One thing that will come up is an explanation of normal conception. The twins know all about their own beginnings, and in the book Nan Tilton wrote about her *in vitro* experience, there are pictures of the embryos. "They think the top one is Heather and the bottom one is Todd," says Nan. "They think it is a very natural thing." The children have seen the scar on their mother's navel and been told that is where the eggs were retrieved from. They understand their conception but not how other children were created. "I would not be discussing intercourse with them at this level," says Nan. "Maybe we could talk about their conception more honestly and openly because it's just such a technological way of being born. It's easier. There is nothing sexual about it. I would say it's going to be awkward talking about sex. I'm going to have to get into the love part kind of around the back door."

Heather and Todd, the eighteenth and nineteenth children created in the Norfolk *in vitro* clinic, are doing just fine, as could be expected from the tests done at Norfolk several years ago. The twins were then fourteen months old but scored at several months above their age level.

Annette Brodsky, a psychologist at UCLA, has seen studies suggesting that kids born by women who have either been infertile for a long time or had difficulties carrying babies tend to be born with higher I.Q.s

"The children are different in some ways—in a positive direction. The only data we have is that they are given a positive push, intellectually and developmentally." Nobody knows what constitutes the "push"—there are so many variables—but, says Brodsky, "Somebody actually suggested it was the extra hormones given to these women that gave them a boost."

"Medically, these [IVF] kids are okay," says Dorothy Greenfeld, a social worker at the Yale University School of Medicine. "My sense of it, from all the kids I know, is that they're pretty much like other kids."

Greenfeld hypothesizes that if there are any differences, they are the result of the parents' struggle with infertility more than of the method of their conception.

"I would be really interested in seeing if these couples are more protective," she says. "The parents of these precious babies may be saying to themselves, 'God, this is the thing we worked for for ten years. Do we dare get angry? Do we dare? How could I even think about wanting to dump this kid on somebody for a day?' "

Nan Tilton does not admit to being overprotective but does concede, "I was very protective in the sense that I didn't just go off and leave them." The first time she and her husband left the twins, they were well prepared. "I hired two nannies to stay, and I had my mother check in every day. We called every day, and I even set up play dates with other women. It was real overkill. I needed that in order to leave."

Five thousand *in vitro* and GIFT babies have been born all over the world, most, according to Hodgen, in the past twenty-four months. Even China, with its strict population control measures, is getting into the act. *In vitro* fertilization, although still the last choice, is now a standard procedure. Only the implantation stage still baffles the doctors. While research is trying to perfect that tricky step, alternatives to the *in vitro* process are also being developed.

Embryo Transfer

The Seed brothers, Richard, a physicist, and Randolph, a surgeon, of Fertility and Genetics Research, Inc. (FGR) in Chicago are hoping to go into big business with a new procedure, embryo transfer. Also referred to as "adoptive pregnancy," it is a technique that has been adapted from cattle breeding. The Seed brothers have linked up with Dr. John Buster of UCLA's Reproductive Endocrinology Unit and Memorial Health Technologies of Long Beach, California (a for-profit subsidiary of the not-for-profit Memorial Health Services), and they have the backing of some private investors, among them Mr. Larry Suscy, a Chicago investment banker who is also the chairman of FGR.

What is being done in cattle, and now in women, is flushing an embryo from the womb of one female and transferring it to the womb of another.

"There is nothing new in all this. It's all very feasible. It's just a case of setting it up," says Dr. Buster. "You understand it is done in the cattle business all the time."[15]

Indeed, Richard Seed is the founder of a cattle breeding company, and in the production of championship cattle, embryo transfer is working very well—not so much to the delight of the cows, who have to suffer a fair amount of discomfort, but to that of their owners. Embryo transfer in cattle produces not only fine animals, but $32 million in yearly revenues for various breeding corporations.

"I don't mind telling you that I expect to get a Nobel Prize," Richard Seed said in a 1980 interview,[16] but that has not been awarded to him yet, although FGR has produced thirteen pregnancies and eleven human births.

"We've lost six million dollars pursuing research and getting this established," says Suscy. The government refused to fund the company's research and investors were skeptical of the profit potential.

"Suscy had to compete for the same [investor] dollars that are normally spread into oil and gas and gold," says Buster. "That's hard competition, because the investors don't care really what you're doing. They just want to be sure to get the money back.''[17] Nevertheless, Suscy succeeded in raising enough money to get started.

The technique that FGR is trying to turn into a profit-making procedure ''is based on the fundamental biological phenomenon that any mammal of the same species can carry an embryo of that species,'' says Suscy. ''The recovery procedure is a fairly normal ob/gyn thing. The transfer is brand-new.''

This is how it is supposed to work.

The essential players are two women—one fertile and one infertile—who ovulate in synchrony and have similar physical characteristics, hair color, height, etc. At the time of ovulation, the fertile woman is artificially inseminated with the sperm of the barren woman's husband, a simple procedure. She then goes home. Five days later she returns to the physician's office, where 60 cc. (approximately two ounces) of a nutrient fluid is pumped into her uterus. If she has conceived, the fertilized egg, which is now an embryo, will be resting—still unattached—on the uterine wall. The fluid flushes it out and into a special catheter. This process is called ''lavage.''

In the laboratory the lavage fluid is transferred to a dish and placed on the heated stage of a microscope. With a high-resolution lens, the lab technician searches out the colorless sphere of 80 to 100 cells, the embryo. Once located, it is photographed and put in a transfer medium and then sucked into a catheter.

The catheter is run up through the cervix of the barren woman, and the embryo is injected into her uterus. If everything goes well, it will implant itself in her uterine lining and grow there for nine months, then the barren woman will give birth to a child that is genetically related to her husband but not to her. The child's biological mother is the egg donor.

Julie and Robert Bradford of California had a baby through the program. They do not know who the biological mother is. She had been selected from respondents to a newspaper ad, had been screened psychologically and medically, and was paid $50 per uterine lavage and a $200 bonus when the fertilized egg was recovered.[18]

The Bradfords are delighted with this method of conception, and there are other enthusiasts.

''I like the simplicity of it. It is noninvasive and that's the big difference,'' says Dr. Evelyn Karson, an obstetrician and a senior staff fellow at the National Institutes of Health. ''Why should a woman have a needle stuck in her belly when her husband can inseminate a woman and have the embryo recovered? When there is a genetic defect—and there are a huge number of defects that are X-linked, passed down only by the woman's genes—the woman can borrow an egg from somebody else. That's one advantage I can see."

Even though embryo transfer eliminates surgery, it is still invasive for the egg donor, and the procedure has several drawbacks. One is the extremely low success rate at all levels of the procedure. In 1983 Dr. Maria Bustillo, a doctor formerly on the transfer team, reported to a group of scientists that "in twenty-five lavage sequences, eleven ova were recovered on the first lavage. That is a recovery rate of forty-four percent. One donor from whom an ova [sic] was not recovered had a retained pregnancy which she spontaneously aborted." Seven of the eleven recovered eggs were found in various stages of insufficient development, ranging from six to fourteen cells. One was degenerate. Only "two well-formed blastocysts were recovered and led to two ongoing pregnancies," Dr. Bustillo told the audience.[19]

In 1984 the recovery rate was twenty-five embryos in fifty-two flushings, but there have still only been eleven births since FGR went into business.

Without much statistical human evidence to go on, Dr. Buster and Dr. Bustillo, who had to come up with more encouraging news if FGR was to stay in business, computed a mathematical model that relies on embryo transfer data not only in humans but also in cattle, monkeys, and baboons. The projections based on this zoo suggest, according to the doctors, that once the donor pool is large enough to assure an entering recipient that she will be matched every time she ovulates, her chances of getting pregnant range from one in twenty to as high as one in three.

These are pie-in-the-sky figures so far, not only because the procedure has not been perfected, but also because the enormous donor pool is not available. Richard Seed, however, has a vision of how it can be worked out. "We try to set up a system similar to a blood bank's, in which every recipient must provide one or two donors for the egg bank."[20]

And says Dr. Buster, "I hope that by operating multiple clinics in the country, we can have a thousand donors available all the time. That means that a recipient woman walking into any clinic in the nation will not only know there's a good chance she'll get an egg that month, but that it will come from a lady who looks just like her and has good genetics."[21]

"We know they [the egg donors] are out there, that there are thousands of them," Buster conjectures.[22] But even if there are fertile women willing to help infertile ones, they may back off when they hear about the high risks for low pay. Whereas the danger to the recipient is virtually nil, the donor runs the same risks of impairment as any woman who has an abortion. In addition, if the physician fails to flush out the embryo, she may have to live with an unwanted pregnancy or submit to a standard abortion procedure. An even greater danger if the embryo is not recovered is an ectopic pregnancy, which could happen if the embryo is flushed up the oviduct during lavage.

"That is one of the major hazards," concedes Dr. Jaroslav Hulka of the International Embryo Transfer Society. "So far, I think it's uniquely human. I don't think the cow has ectopic pregnancies. That's one of the worrisome aspects of trying to take a technology developed in one species and apply it to another."[23]

FGR envisions that eventually the donor-recipient matching will be done by a computer storing information from all over the country. It is a grand scheme, but the field is already crowded with reproductive services. In 1986 FGR set up several centers but had to close them down because of other competitive technologies, namely IVF and GIFT.

"I wouldn't say competitive, I would say overlapping technologies," Suscy insists. "It made us realize that what the patients need, what they benefit from, are centers where all the techniques and technologies are offered side by side with high quality. To have solely embryo transfer—that wasn't going to meet the market."

"The way I'd like to see it organized is as an ancillary department of a hospital open to the community," says Michael Eberhard, vice president of Memorial Health Technologies. "It would be provided as a service to obstetricians. It's not controlled by a medical group, not even controlled by a hospital. Any doctor can refer their patient to it."[24]

FGR is adapting to survive. It is currently licensing embryo transfer technology to hospital and medical groups.

Who are the potential patients who would benefit from embryo transfer?

FGR estimates that at least 50,000 women would be eligible for the procedure each year. But at the moment "adoptive pregnancy" is in direct competition with the better established IVF and GIFT technologies, regardless of what Mr. Suscy says. Embryo transfer has the advantage of not requiring surgery or heavy drug treatments, but the cost is approximately the same as *in vitro* and GIFT. The major disadvantage, in the eyes of many people, is that the mother does not give birth to her own genetic child.

Women who are carriers of genetic diseases may prefer to borrow an egg from somebody else. "If you take a woman with cystic fibrosis or a carrier of hemophelia and she says, 'I choose not to have my own; I prefer to borrow an egg from you; I will have borne it and I feel safe,' that individual choice repeated again and again will totally eliminate those diseases," Suscy explains optimistically. "That's what has excited us and kept us going. The infertility is sixty percent, and the genetics, forty percent."

But even in the area of genetic screening, embryo transfer faces competition from IVF, which will soon be able to screen the embryo for chromosomal abnormalities before it is put back in the uterus, and preconception sex selection, which is becoming somewhat more reliable, will more easily be able to eliminate gender-linked genetic diseases.

Where embryo transfer has a unique potential corner of the market is as a therapy for women who cannot produce an egg, either because they have been born without ovaries, had them destroyed by disease or surgery, or where they simply do not function properly. A woman with malfunctioning ovaries but with a healthy uterus may not produce the hormones necessary to sustain a pregnancy, but such hormones could be supplied by the doctor.

FGR has not yet achieved a pregnancy in an anovarian woman (a woman without ovaries), but they are working on it. If they manage, they may well be able to extend childbearing age to women past their normal childbearing age. Even there, though, they have been nosed out by a South African team who transferred an embryo conceived *in vitro* into the womb of the egg donor's forty-eight-year-old mother. The four-foot-eleven-inch ninety-eight-pound grandmother gave birth to her own grandchildren—triplets.

Ovum Transfer

Norfolk has done about forty "ovum transfers," an IVF-related procedure that involves a woman donating just an egg. The egg is fertilized in a dish with the sperm from another woman's husband, then implanted into that woman. Ten pregnancies and six births have occurred at Norfolk through use of this technique, and this may be the largest such donor program in the country.

What are the risks of carrying an unrelated embryo?

"None," says Dr. Gary Hodgen. "We wondered about that. We took rhesus monkeys that had no ovaries for three or more years—some for as many as eleven. I gave them estrogen and progesterone in a manner imaging what the ovaries would do in a normal ovarian menstrual cycle. That causes the endometrium to grow. Then we put embryos in from other monkeys genetically unrelated. They carried them to term; they had normal babies. Not only did they carry them well, but their pregnancy rate was high. I couldn't believe it. The year after that, the first woman was done in Melbourne, Australia, then six in Israel, two more in Europe, and there were four or five here—now, around the world, thirty or forty. So the pregnancy rate is high; the kids are normal. We just dropped our concern in the face of that evidence.''

In June 1987 Dr. Martin Quigley of the Cleveland Clinic announced that his hospital was setting up an anonymous egg donor program. The ''adopting'' couple pays $1200 for the egg donor's participation. The hospital was reportedly ''deluged with people who want to donate eggs.''[25]

''The limitation is the availability of donors,'' says Dr. Zev Rosenwaks, who started the ovum transfer program at Norfolk. ''For the first three years, I can tell you I did it all myself to the last drop, with some assistance from fellows.''

Egg donors are sometimes IVF patients who have given up excess eggs; others are perfectly fertile women who have planned to have a tubal ligation and are willing to have their ovaries stimulated beforehand to produce extra eggs.

Similar to sperm donation, the ovum transfer program matches egg donor to recipient in terms of hair color, eye color, height, etc. And similar to sperm donation, the parties do not meet.

Some sisters have donated eggs but, according to Rosenwaks, ''We prefer that they not be sisters. We would rather they be anonymous, for the same reason that sperm donation is anonymous. We are dealing, at least from a legal, social point of view, in a new area. The difficulty is not with the technical aspects of this procedure, but are there going to be emotional problems, social problems, legal problems, in terms of identity, in terms of ownership? We do have donors sign an agreement that says once they give up the egg, they've given up ownership. For the actual couple who receives the egg, what they do in terms of telling their child is really up to them.''

Unlike sperm donors, egg donors, at least at Norfolk—and by recommendation of the American Fertility Society—are not paid. Their motivation, according to Rosenwaks, is ''altruistic.''

''I believe there should be compensation for the time they spend—they lose work time. They should be compensated in a reasonable way, but I don't think it should be exorbitant fees that will create an inducement for donation, which would bring up the question of whether you are selling something for profit.''

Although advertising may be necessary in the future, Rosenwaks does not like the idea.

"It's a very private thing to donate an egg. We prefer that physicians in the area discuss it with their patients—tell them, 'You're going to have a tubal ligation anyway; what do you think about making a donation?' That would be ideal. Practically, it might be that in the future we'll have to advertise. It is a problem getting donors. On the other hand, what happens if someone comes in and they're not that healthy and we make a judgment that they shouldn't? Well, you have problems there. There are some problems that come along with advertising that we haven't been willing to deal with. . . . We'd like to keep it private, and low-key.''

But ovum transfer raises even more complex questions about who the mother is.

Norfolk's Dr. Rosenwaks notes that "technically, biologically" the egg donor is the genetic mother because it is her genetic material. But the *biological* mother, in this case the woman who carries the child and who wants the child, is viewed as the official mother by the medical establishment.

Rosenwaks says there is no problem carrying a genetically unrelated baby. "Remember, the father, who has half the genetic material in any pregnancy, is antigenic. He's foreign to the mother. So the mother is carrying a child that to her is foreign anyway. This just represents two doses instead of one.''

Should Government Fund Research?

While the new technologies have brought hope to many, some people worry that the procedures are too heavily weighted toward the profit motive. There is an unavoidable suspicion that the new "fixes" are not so much for the good of the infertile as for the financial good of the entrepreneurs, some of whom are patenting not only their tools, but their procedures.

"Ordinarily when you develop a new medical procedure, it's reported in the scientific literature and, if it has merit, it receives wide dissemination,'' B. J. Anderson, associate general counsel for the American Medical Association told Gena Corea, author of the *Mother Machine*. "You don't attempt to commercialize it and limit it to a few in order to gain economic advantage.''[26]

Replies Suscy of FGR, "You know what? There is this incredible hypocrisy about the whole thing. In the reproductive field, everybody is filing for patents like mad." According to Suscy, at least fifty medical procedures have already been patented in the past. (FGR itself has sought to patent both the leak-free devices developed for the embryo retrieval and the retrieval procedure.)

The National Institutes of Health's Dr. Evelyn Karson blames the government for the commercialism that threatens to dominate reproductive technology. "The government has refused to fund research like that, and this is what happens. Why is all of this going on in the private sector? Because somebody has to pay for it, and if people are willing to gamble and pay for it, well, fine. This country has made the decision that it would rather spend its money on guns, so there is only one alternative: Either we stop dead in our tracks or we let these entrepreneurs go ahead and do it."

"It is not as if the government is giving out money," says Anne Kranz, a member of Resolve. "There is very little research in the area of infertility compared with either mental illness or cancer of whatever; it's minuscule. We keep hoping for more major research."

Whether or not the government should fund research in the area of infertility is, of course, debatable. Infertile couples constitute a small minority of the population, and society as a whole will not suffer any ill effects from their failure to reproduce. Although pundits like Ben Wattenberg, author of the *Birth Dearth*, see a bleak future for the Western world if its white middle class does not breed more prolifically, there are enough children born in this country to keep population numbers up. It is easy to argue that the government's first priority ought to be on research into cures for common deadly diseases and a more equitable distribution of medical services.

Infertility is nevertheless a serious problem—a problem, one is often led to believe, that afflicts mainly the white middle class. Those who smile with their miracle offspring from the pages of new magazines are generally well-educated and well-off people who have the intellectual and financial wherewithal to know what options are available and to pursue them to the end of the line. The Washington, D.C., branch of Resolve conducted a survey of its members and found that an astonishing 94 percent had college degrees, and a full two-thirds had graduate degrees. The infertile couples that we read about in the newspapers and see on TV when a baby has been created by some astonishing procedure are invariably vocal, well-educated, and well-heeled people. We never hear about the vast majority of childless couples who struggle on or give up in total anonymity. They remain faceless statistics.

Infertility and Capitalism

"Like it or not," says Dr. Stillman, "a capitalistic society runs on a free marketplace. People who have more money will have more ability to buy a car, and therefore can get around more easily—and maybe get more jobs because they can get around. They have more ability to survive a heart attack because they get an ambulance more quickly to their house, which is located in a nice neighborhood where the police will answer the phone quicker. It goes on and on. The rich get richer. The same thing that occurs for medical care is true in treating infertility. In this country it is not a matter of suppressing economically disadvantaged people; it is only that those who have some economic advantage will have the purely financial means by which to take advantage of the services. Is that fair? I don't say it is fair, I'm saying that's the system in which we live."

It is a sad fact that some people with infertility problems cannot have children because they do not have enough money for treatment, but that should not prevent those couples who have the means to pursue happiness from doing so. However, the inequities place society in an uncomfortable moral situation. While the health care system allows the wealthy to conjure up babies out of petri dishes, the same system affords little care to poor infants who have been conceived without medical intervention. While miracle babies are treated as precious symbols of our technical know-how and advancing civilization, thousands of poor babies die due to the lack of adequate care. Infant mortality rates in the United States are among the highest in the developed world. The babies who die in infancy are mostly minority poor, and maternal deaths follow the same pattern.

Says Wendy Chavkin, director of the Bureau of Maternity Services and Family Planning for the city of New York, "In the United States there are great disparities in the rate women die in association with pregnancy. There is a strong association with no prenatal care and maternal death, and with poverty and race; the association is very strong. In fact, we haven't had a white maternal death in New York the last few years. We have about thirty-five a year, mostly Hispanic and black."

"It is terribly offensive," says ethicist John Fletcher. "What you are looking at is a contradiction in society. The United States is loaded with contradictions. There is a limit to what a society can take before it has a corporate vomiting and says, 'This is too repulsive.' "

As individuals we do not really think we are being socially irresponsible by having expensive, scientifically conceived children while at the same time many children do not get the most basic care. But switch the scene to India, for example. Shock is not an uncommon response to the news that India, with its armies of homeless, begging children, is nevertheless creating *in vitro* babies. Indians are no different from Americans, it appears, when it comes to the problem of children. If it is shocking that India creates test tube babies when so many children go wanting, it is no less shocking in the United States.

It is strange to think that infertile people who have a simple and natural wish for children are the ones who fuel entrepreneurs' money-making schemes, who make and break the reputations of doctors, who make the rest of us nervous about reducing life to chemical recipes. All they want is a baby. It is all they think about. Only the rare infertile couple gives any thought to the wider political and ethical problems they have helped create along with babies. As long as they cannot have their desired offspring by normal means, they are going to push for new technologies that can fulfill their wishes regardless of the consequences for the rest of society. And if science and medicine fail the infertile woman, she still may not give up on her dream. She may ask other women to help her.

6

Surrogate Motherhood

IN THE WORLD'S OLDEST PROFESSION, A WOMAN'S BODY IS FOR hire; in the newest it is, too.

Attorney Noel P. Keane's Dearborn, Michigan, office is teeming with young women in search of customers for a cooperative venture that involves no sex but does involve pregnancy and a good deal of money. The customers, who have flown in from distant places, are well-groomed, respectable-looking people unable to have a child of their own. The young women, who are offering to loan their wombs to the couples, bounce babies on their knees as proof of their fertility and quality offspring. Some of them are accompanied by male companions who testify to their woman's ability as breeders. The couples are assigned private offices, and the hopeful young mothers make their rounds and look happy or dejected as they come out of their interviews.

Noel Keane is there to clinch the deal; he is in the baby business. He links up infertile couples with women who will be impregnated with the sperm of a husband, not their own, and turn the child that they bear over to the sperm donor and his infertile wife. Welcome to the world of surrogacy.

Like a problem one hopes will go away if ignored, the practice

127

of surrogacy occupied the dim outer reaches of the public consciousness for almost a decade. "It was seen as a sort of fringe thing that very few people would want to get involved with," says George J. Annas, professor of Health Law at the Boston University School of Medicine. ". . . a lot of people just thought it would go away . . . That appears not to be the case."[1]

Surrogacy is not a new phenomenon, it has biblical precedents. In the book of Genesis we are told that Abraham's wife, Sarah, wanted a child but could not have one, so she had a slave woman, Hagar, "lie with" Abraham and a son, Ishmael, was born. However, Hagar became uppity as a result of her new role and was banned along with the child. Ishmael became the founder of the lost tribe through which Islam claims Abrahamic ancestry. Later on in Genesis another childless woman, Rachel, the wife of Jacob, used the services of a surrogate slave woman, Bilhah; and Rachel's sister, Leah, who had several children of her own, decided after she lost her fecundity to have still more children, and her slave woman Zilpah gave her two sons. At the risk of being slightly irreverent, one might even say that God himself used a surrogate, and a virgin at that, to have his only son, Jesus Christ.

But in spite of hallowed precedents, surrogacy, which has probably been practiced in the deepest secrecy ever since biblical times, was not seen as a socially acceptable way to compensate for a wife's infertility. Nevertheless, ever since Noel Keane got involved in surrogacy in 1976, the practice has crept slowly but inexorably into open practice. It is estimated that about 600 surrogate babies have been born in the United States in the last decade. Noel Keane alone has arranged close to 200 surrogate births.

Although from the very beginning, Noel Keane used the "Phil Donahue Show" almost as a personal publicity platform, appearing on television several times with couples and surrogates to acquaint a rapt, top-rated Nielsen audience with the ins and outs of surrogacy, the general public paid the practice little attention until the Baby M case hit front pages across the country.

The vast majority of surrogate arrangements have worked out to the satisfaction of both infertile couples and surrogates, but inasmuch as surrogacy started out in a social, legal, and emotional no man's land, sooner or later something was bound to go wrong. The Baby M case was not the first instance of a surrogacy conflict. From the beginning there were horror stories, such as a surrogate mother extorting money from an infertile couple and giving birth to a baby with drug withdrawal symptoms, but there have also been touching examples of true altruism and lifelong mutually respectful relationships. The Baby M case, however, "really brought to the hilt every single terror of not being able to count on what is going to happen when the baby is born," says Constance Shapiro.

The story of Baby M started out like any other surrogate birth. Mary Beth Whitehead, twenty-nine, the wife of a garbage collector and the mother of two, agreed to be inseminated with the sperm of William Stern, forty-one, a professor of biochemistry, and to turn the child over to Mr. Stern immediately after its birth. William Stern's wife, Elizabeth, forty-one, a professor of pediatrics, has a self-diagnosed mild case of multiple sclerosis that she believes would be aggravated by pregnancy, and she therefore chose not to bear her own children. Through attorney Noel P. Keane's "branch office," the Infertility Institute in New York City, Whitehead and the Sterns were brought together. An agreement was worked out and contracts signed. Whitehead was to receive $10,000 in return for her services, the money to be held in escrow until the child was born.

An amicable relationship developed between the two couples. They talked regularly on the phone, and the Sterns invited twelve-year-old Ryan Whitehead to a baseball game, and William Stern and Mary Beth Whitehead drove to New York together for the inseminations. The Whiteheads' daughter spent a night with the Sterns and went to the Macy's Thanksgiving Day Parade with them. As the pregnancy progressed, however, Mary Beth began to get annoyed with the Sterns for interfering in her life. William Stern, for instance, would call Mary Beth's doctor and recommend drugs that she should take. Even before the baby was born, Whitehead began to wish she had never gotten into the arrangement and began to have doubts about her ability to relinquish the baby. She asked the Sterns to be allowed to visit the baby, and they agreed, as long as she agreed to remain anonymous.

On March 27, 1986, Whitehead gave birth to a baby girl whom she called Sarah; on March 30 she relinquished the child to the Sterns. However, she missed the baby and persuaded the Sterns to let her keep the child for a week. She nursed the child and decided to keep her. Refusing to accept the $10,000, Whitehead informed the Sterns of her decision. To keep the Sterns, who wanted the baby back, at arm's length or more, Whitehead fled with her family to her mother's home in Florida on May 6. While in Florida, she talked on the phone with the Sterns, who begged her to let them have the baby. Whitehead threatened to kill herself and the baby if the Sterns tried to take the baby away from her. Eighty-seven days later the police seized the child and brought her back to New Jersey, and a court order granted the Sterns temporary custody of the baby, whom they called Melissa. Whitehead was accorded twice-weekly visitation rights. Mr. Stern brought suit against Whitehead for breach of contract, and on January 5, 1987, the trial opened in Bergen County Superior Court. For weeks the whole country stood by as experts testified, journalists scribbled, members of the Committee for Mary Beth Whitehead and Mothers with Feelings demonstrated, and the judge prepared for a verdict. On March 31 Harvey R. Sorkow, the judge in the case, upheld the surrogate contract, gave custody of the child, always referred to as Baby M during the trial, to the Sterns, and immediately after the verdict allowed Mrs. Stern to adopt the baby. Mary Beth Whitehead's rights to the child were thereby terminated.

The trial was ugly. Most of the venom was directed at Mary Beth Whitehead. She was adjudged too enmeshed with her own children because she spent too much time braiding her daughter's hair, and she was a bad mother because she said "hooray" instead of "pat-a-cake" when her child clapped her hands. She was deemed narcissistic because she dyed her hair, called emotionally unstable, and told the family environment was unhealthy because her husband had had trouble with alcohol. The fact that the financial affairs of the Whiteheads were not in the best of condition was also cited against them. The Sterns, on the other hand, were portrayed as a loving couple and stable citizens.

The contract dispute turned into a custody battle with an unprecedented outcome. The biological mother of the child was deprived of visitation rights without any real proof that she was an unfit mother.

The trial hit a nerve in the U.S. public, and the case was endlessly debated in the press. A grim-looking Mary Beth, surrounded by her family and holding a picture of her Sarah, stared from the front cover of the *New York Times Sunday Magazine*, and every publication, from the *Wall Street Journal* to sensational tabloids, had an opinion piece on surrogate motherhood and interviews with anyone who claimed special insight into the phenomenon.

Although *Newsweek* opinion polls taken at the time of Judge Sorkow's verdict found that the majority of the general public thought his decision correct, most of the articles that appeared about the case were tinged with a sense of horror, not only about the treatment of Mary Beth Whitehead in court but also about surrogacy itself. There were charges of baby-selling. Feminists attacked surrogacy as a new form of exploitation of women. Class differences between the surrogate and the couple were brought up as proof that economically disadvantaged women would turn into a herd of breeders for wealthy people. And everyone was caught in the dilemma of deciding where the child's best interests lay. Several "experts" called for a ban on surrogacy, and most everybody else advocated that it be regulated by law.

The Baby M case certainly demonstrated that a surrogate arrangement can turn into a horror story. It was definitely a worst case scenario, but it was not the whole story.

A surrogacy arrangement is a complicated and potentially risky business. The drama of bringing a surrogate baby into the world stars an infertile couple and a surrogate mother and features a large supporting cast of surrogate agencies, doctors, lawyers, and psychologists. The child, the most important character, shines by its absence, but everything revolves around it—the child creates the plot. The denouement is unpredictable, and nobody knows until the child has been adopted whether they are actors in a heartwarming drama or in a tragedy of errors.

A New Hope for Infertile Couples

The gas tank was on Empty, and they got lost on the way to the hospital for the birth of their baby. They stopped to ask a forest ranger for directions. "Oh gee," he said. "That hospital is so far away that I don't even know where it is." So they had a big argument. As the tension mounted Carol Wright, thirty-four, yelled at her husband, Peter, thirty-six, for not having had the gas tank filled up, while Peter accused Carol of not getting good directions.

At the hospital Dee Perry, thirty-two, had everything under control. Her husband Dale, thirty-five, was there with her. She had had labor induced at 8 o'clock, but nothing much had happened by the time Carol and Peter stumbled in at 9:30 A.M. They did not miss the birth of their son, Matthew.

It is a bit confusing, but all four people played a vital role in the life of the baby who was born that same afternoon, January 8, 1987, at 3:35.

Carol, a teacher, is infertile because her mother took DES (diethylstilbestrol), a drug widely prescribed in the 1950s for the prevention of miscarriage. Only years later was it discovered that it often caused infertility and a predisposition to certain cancers in the next generation. Carol had been married for twelve years when, after many operations and tests, the doctors finally told her that she would never get pregnant. She was in despair.

"It sounds a little traditional," she says, "but having a baby is the ultimate fulfillment of being a woman, and not to be able to have one makes you feel abnormal."

"It was very sad," says Peter. "It's like losing a child you've known all along."

They tried to adopt, but there were no newborn white babies available. Then one day Carol read a story on surrogate motherhood in a news magazine.

"I didn't think much about it," says Carol, "but a few days later, I just woke up and looked at myself in the mirror and said, 'That's perfect.' "

Her husband, vice-president of an advertising agency in Massachusetts, felt it was a little strange—they did not know anybody who had ever had a surrogate baby—and was not really sure it was possible, but he was nevertheless "delighted" with the idea.

"When Carol came through with this, I knew it was the answer. I could see in her eyes how excited she was that this was the right way for us."

Carol called the Hagar Institute in Kansas, the only licensed surrogacy agency in the United States. According to founder Beth Bacon, thirty-eight, a former social worker specializing in adoption, it is run very much like an adoption agency.

"When I heard about surrogacy, I was initially as shocked as everybody else," says Bacon, "but the more I thought about it, the more I felt it could be a wonderful thing—and it could be a disaster." She opened her agency in Topeka, Kansas, in 1982, and although a few of her friends "were hysterical" at the thought, most people were simply very curious about surrogacy. "I have rarely run into anybody who was dead against it," she says.

The Hagar Institute sent Carol and Peter a tape explaining how the agency got started and what the surrogate process was all about. Feeling a bit like pioneers, they were reassured by "a nice, Midwestern, down-to-earth, homespun voice."

In Missouri, Dee had listened to the same tape, and so had her husband, Dale, who owns a refrigeration business. Dee had heard about the Hagar Institute through her gynecologist, and when she later saw one of their ads for surrogates in the local paper, she proposed the idea of becoming a surrogate to her husband.

"I thought she was pulling my leg," says Dale. "I knew little about the surrogate program, and I was kind of shocked. Most

people are, I think, when they get firsthand news of surrogacy face
to face."

But Dee, who has made motherhood her principal role in life,
was serious. She had already given birth to a boy, now four, and a
girl, two.

"I enjoyed being pregnant and had babies very easily. Both of
my deliveries were very quick," said Dee. "I just like having
babies. A close friend of mine—I have known her since second
grade—cannot have children, so there was a little motivation there
looking at her. I enjoy my own children, and after looking at how
many infertile couples there are out there, I thought it was definitely something I wanted to do."

Dale decided to be supportive.

As a surrogate candidate, Dee had to go through a lot of medical
and psychological evaluations required by the Hagar Institute. The
agency also sends out a social worker to do home studies of both
the surrogate and the childless couple. Dee "put her best foot
forward" in the four-hour long conversation with the representative from the institute.

"The main thing we look for," says Bacon, "is emotional
stability and physical health. We look for a woman who is mature
and understands what she is doing. She must be over twenty-one
and have a good, healthy lifestyle."

Only one in seventeen applicants are accepted into the program,
but Dee had the right qualities, so she was signed up.

Two days before Christmas 1985, the social worker arrived in
Boston to evaluate Peter and Carol. They wanted to make a good
impression.

"I'm pretty neat, so I wasn't worried about that, but I did bake
blueberry muffins that morning," says Carol.

"We were very nervous," says Peter. "We knew we had to be
accepted into the program to do this, and we thought the standards
were so high we would never qualify."

"We're not looking for the perfect parents," says Bacon, "but
we want to make sure that they seem like stable people and that
their marriage and adjustment to infertility, as well as their attitude
to surrogate mothers, are okay. We certainly don't want anyone in
the program who thinks that surrogates are just a bunch of money-
grubbing, low-life people, because they will pass that on to the
child, and the child must have positive feelings about his origin."

"It was the first face-to-face contact," says Carol, "and actually we enjoyed it very much. The social worker was extremely

professional and pleasant, and we had an enjoyable interview and exchange of information.

"We had made up our minds before she came, that if we were right for the program, we were going to do it."

So they signed the contract with the Hagar Institute, and the social worker left with a big check—the whole program cost about $25,000 and $8,500 of that was the surrogate mother's fee.

"The whole process is scary, that's for sure," says Carol. "You're committing yourself to a lot of money and a risk of sorts. The money is out there regardless of whether you ever have a child. That's scary, and the emotional risk is equally scary, but we felt it was our big chance to have a family."

"For us it was the end of a long phase. We were a little bit nervous, but we were incredibly excited, and we felt fortunate that we could afford it," says Peter.

They had to remortgage their house to come up with the money.

The Legal Foreplay

Anita Cody, thirty-nine, and her husband, Bart, a dentist in the Baltimore area, signed up with Infertility Associates International in Chevy Chase, Maryland, after a talk with the director, Harriet Blankfeld, in her office.

"We are not an adoption agency," Blankfeld says, "so we don't go to somebody's house and measure their rooms and interview them there. But the material information we get is quality information. We know they are psychologically well, we know they have the ability to parent, and we know why they want to go through this."

Anita suffers from unexplained infertility, has had one ectopic pregnancy, and tried *in vitro* without any luck.

"I don't think there is any procedure I didn't have," says Anita. "I think I shed enough tears over the years."

The Codys had adopted a boy through Baltimore County Special Services in 1980 and wanted a sibling for their son. Special Services gave them a daughter, but then the biological mother changed her mind.

"So we sent the baby back," says Anita. "We really didn't want to go through that again, so at that point we decided to go with something safer, which was to try a surrogate program. The biological factor was not as important as knowing that we had a better shot at keeping this baby."

The paper is pink, but the language written on it corresponds to its size—legal. The pastel document from Infertility Associates International reads in places: "A surrogate mother . . . shall be impregnated via artificial insemination of the sperm of the father. The surrogate mother shall carry the baby to term and upon the baby's birth shall be delivered to the parents." Rule 5 in the contract stipulates "that the father must be willing to collect and deliver his sperm specimens to the treating physician as specified by the treating physician when requested and as often as needed— failure to do so may be considered a breach of contract." It also says, ". . . upon the delivery of the baby to the parents and in return for that said delivery and for the service of the pregnancy and the delivery of the baby, the surrogate mother receives her fee . . . for this service, of Ten Thousand Dollars." Underlined in a rather disheartening way, a sentence cautions the future parents, *"It is understood that these rights and liabilities may or may not be honored in a Court of Law should a breach arise."*

With addenda, the contract is thirteen pages long, but in spite of the detailed rules and regulations and the possible presence of lawyers at the signing, the contract may not be worth the pink paper it is printed on. The first test of the validity of a surrogate contract was the Baby M case, and the judge upheld it. However, other judges are not bound to follow the New Jersey precedent. Nevertheless, reading and signing this document of uncertain value is the kind of legal foreplay that took place before the conception of Annie Gallo, who was born in the late fall of 1985.

Annie's mother, Lorna, a thirty-two-year-old hairdresser who works out of her home in New Jersey, had tried for eight years to get pregnant. She had chronic endometriosis and went through seven surgeries before she had a hysterectomy in 1980 that ended her dreams of having a child of her own. Even before her hysterectomy, she was on an adoption list, but then she got divorced. Her husband "already had a son from a previous marriage and didn't really care that I couldn't get pregnant or had a hysterectomy," says Lorna, "so right after my hysterectomy, I left him, making a clean slate of it." She got married again to Mitchell, an inventory supervisor, and let the adoption agency know. The agency dropped her name to the bottom of the list.

Lorna sank into depression and went into therapy. Her new husband "didn't desperately want children," but when he heard about a surrogacy agency on the radio, he came home and told her about it to cheer her up. They made an appointment with Infertility

Associates International. Lorna used her divorce settlement to pay for the fees.

When infertile couples turn to surrogacy, they are usually at the end of the line. They have gone through countless medical procedures and have already spent considerable amounts of money in pursuit of a baby. Not wanting to give up hope, they have pursued medical solutions for years, often so long that by the time they begin to look into adoption, they are too old to be considered. For many adoption agencies the cut-off age is thirty-five. And adoption agencies always suffer a shortage of healthy, white infants.

Economic Considerations of Surrogacy

Marilyn Smith, thirty-six, who lives in Missouri with her second husband, a house painter, also had a hysterectomy and also tried adoption, but "it was a hopeless thing. After four years we kind of gave up on it." But Marilyn would not give up on having a baby, "so that's why we ended up doing it this way," meaning surrogacy. Marilyn also signed up with the Hagar Institute and paid what was for her a very large sum of money.

"We are not rich people," says Marilyn. "We saved for three years for this money. We are just basic blue-collar workers. It's month to month, you know—'Oh, look how much the electric bill is!' We saved and scrimped and it was difficult for us to come up with that much money."

Critics of surrogacy often bring up class differences between surrogates and the couples for whom they bear children. They fear that surrogacy will create a class of underprivileged baby breeders. Says Barbara Katz Rothman, a sociologist at the City University of New York and Baruch College, "We need to have a public policy to address the very real problem of infertility, but not by allowing rich people to use poor women to bear their children for them."[2]

There is no doubt that couples who have surrogate babies tend to be better off than the surrogates themselves, but the differences are generally not as stark as presumed. As John Robertson, professor of law at the University of Texas, points out, "On the class bias issue, it's not clear that there will be as much class bias as some feminists think. . . . The bottom line is, even if there is a class bias here, it is no different than the class biases that run throughout society. It's all right to hire poor women to be nannies and to do child rearing, [so] why is it not all right to hire them as surrogates?"[3]

Dennis Harrison, a forensic psychologist who tests both couples and surrogates for Surrogate Motherhood, Inc., in Laurel, Maryland, does not see a consistent wide economic gap between surrogates and the couples for whom they bear children.

"The difference economically is not that far. Most of the couples are not rich. They are usually two-income families, and a lot of surrogates are from two-income families, too."

Lorna and Mitchell Gallo are not rich, and Marilyn Smith and her husband are self-professed blue-collar workers. Both couples were picked at random—they do not represent a statistically valid sample—but they at least indicate that there are glaring exceptions to Rothman's vision of economic disparity.

Choosing a Surrogate

Peter and Carol were "quite exhilarated and excited" when they sat down to look at the dozen or so profiles of surrogates that the social worker from the Hagar Institute had given them.

They chose Dee.

"It was her picture," says Carol. "She had a wholesome, very honest, down-to-earth look about her, and her kids were lovely. We also liked her reason for doing it. She had a friend from childhood who couldn't have children, and she wanted to help somebody else. We liked that. Her medical background looked fine, and her husband was supportive."

In March, without ever having met, Carol and Peter signed a contract with Dee. Most agencies order the husband, who donates sperm for the insemination, to submit to testing for venereal disease and AIDS, and some also require medical proof that he has an adequate sperm count. In April, after having passed the tests, Peter flew to Kansas for the insemination.

"We got a phone call at five in the afternoon from Hagar— 'You absolutely have to be here tomorrow morning at ten.' We didn't think it was going to be that soon," Carol recalls. "He was packing and I was making plane reservations." Twenty minutes later he was out the door. At the airport in Kansas, Peter rented a fancy sports car "so he would feel especially virile on the way to the doctor's office."

It was a Saturday, so the only staff there was the doctor.

When surrogate Dee stepped into the empty office, she paused.

"I kind of stopped for a minute and thought, 'Well, this is it. I'm here to be inseminated with the sperm of a total stranger. Is this in fact something I really want to do?' And, yes, it was. I knew once I got in there how comfortable I felt; I was doing the right thing.''

Peter thought, "This is the magical moment."

He was there fifteen minutes and flew home again. He never saw Dee.

Dee became pregnant on the first try.

The Hagar Institute phoned Carol to tell her the good news of the pregnancy—several people in the office got on the extensions to cheer—and when her husband came home, she told him, "We are going to have a baby!"

Carol starts to cry. "The whole thing is still so emotional," she squeaks out between sobs.

"We were overjoyed. We couldn't believe it had happened on the first try. We actually had somewhere a little beginning of life that was going to be our child," says Peter.

"I bought Peter a little red wagon as a symbol, a present, when we found out, and he bought me a teddy bear," Carol remembers. "I had also gotten a pink and a blue balloon and tied them to the wagon, and that's what we had in our living room for months and months. The blue balloon deflated in about three days; the pink one lasted, so we knew we were going to have a girl."

Every now and then Carol and Peter asked each other, "Do you really believe that this very fortunate and good thing is happening to us?"

To make it all seem more real, Peter and Carol started to acquire baby clothes and toys.

"These things reminded us that in nine months we were going to have a little baby. Everything having to do with this baby became our greatest joy," Peter remembers.

Pregnant Dee was going through the opposite process. "From day one I told myself this was not a child I was going to keep," says Dee. "My husband and I both decided after my daughter was born that two children was enough for us."

"I told Dee that if she decided to change her mind to keep this baby, she was going to have to raise three children without a husband," says Dale and laughs. "This was set in right from the start."

"We thought that once the pregnancy was achieved, we could breathe a sigh of relief, but that was when it heated up and became more stressful," says Carol. "We were so glad that our surrogate was from Kansas City and not some chick from New York. It would have scared us to death. Dee gave us a very different feeling—wholesome."

Lorna Gallo does not really know what made her choose the surrogate she did. She only got one file, which contained a picture of the surrogate when she was eight years old.

"We just had one girl," says Lorna, "and we decided when we got her picture and her report that she was good. She didn't look anything like me."

Anita and Bart Cody went through more files and found one that they liked in particular.

"She was from a large family. We liked that a lot. She happened to come from a very tall family—we are kind of on the short side, but she was ready."

For the Codys the inseminations were not "a totally pleasurable experience, but it was something my husband felt he had to do for both of us," says Anita. "I was part of it. I had to drive down to Washington with the sperm once because he had to go back to work. We both wanted this very very much. It wasn't one or the other."

Marilyn Smith had a very hard time finding a suitable surrogate.

"None of them was what we wanted; they were not what the average couple would accept," she says. "Most of them were low intelligence and maybe one hundred fifty pounds overweight, where you really worry about their health."

It took nine months of picking through files before Marilyn and her husband decided on a thirty-seven-year-old woman married to a divinity student.

Marilyn questioned the agency about the quality of their surrogates and recalls being told that "if they pass the physical and psychological tests, no matter how dumb or smart or fat or skinny, they have to accept them." But she was also told that she "was under no obligation to choose them."

Some future parents have very specific—and sometimes ludicrous—ideas of what they want in a surrogate. Apparently one single man hoped to find a surrogate who combined the looks of Brigitte Bardot with the brains of Eleanor Roosevelt[4] and another potential father wanted one with breasts shaped to his precise specifications.[5]

Agencies tend to reject people with silly requests. "I've turned down couples who said, 'We want someone five feet three inches tall with an I.Q. of one hundred and fifty-six,' " says William Handel of the Center for Surrogate Parenting in Los Angeles. "I don't want to be accused of playing eugenics. I explain to couples that they can try for a surrogate who looks reasonably close to you . . . If you want to go beyond that, this is not the office."[6]

It took nine months for Marilyn to find a surrogate, and it took ten months for the surrogate to get pregnant. The insemination finally succeeded on what was to have been the last try because the surrogate was moving away to Washington State. She had already relocated when the good news came.

"I was real excited and ran outside and told my husband, and he was kind of skeptical. I remember his first words were, 'Don't you think it is a little bit strange that all of a sudden she is pregnant right before she moves? They are just telling us something because she is so far away.' But it was real."

The Relationship Between Couples and Surrogates

Headlines such as "Husband Runs off with Surrogate" have appeared in the *National Enquirer* and other equally stimulating supermarket check-out line literature. To the average reader they tickle the lust for a little sensation, but to a couple in the surrogate process, such headlines stimulate real fears.

Through Noel Keane's office, Carmen Dubois, forty-seven, and her husband, Ted, fifty-four, a real estate broker, had two surrogate babies born almost simultaneously, to different surrogate mothers. Keane usually requires the couples and surrogates to meet. Carmen balked at that. She did not even want her husband to see the surrogates' pictures.

"I just didn't feel confident myself," she says, "and I was a bit jealous."

Carmen, who has a twenty-four-year-old daughter from a previous marriage, was not sure she wanted more children but, aged forty-three at the time of deciding on surrogacy, nevertheless went along with her husband's wishes when it became clear that her tubes were permanently blocked.

For Carmen, it was difficult in the beginning.

"There were a lot of strong feelings, and I wanted to scream. I wanted to tell them I hated every bit of this, and that I didn't want a kid. But I couldn't for the simple reason that if I said what I really felt, naturally nobody would want to give kids to me."

Carmen found her situation humiliating and frustrating, and she was afraid. "It wasn't that he was going to fall in love—at the time I didn't look so bad. What I was concerned about was: Could he possibly consider them as a mate?" Not taking any chances, Carmen, who accompanied her husband on his trips to Michigan for inseminations—"We made a honeymoon out of each and every visit"—is glad now that she met the surrogates, and she became very close to one of them.

Dennis Harrison, a forensic psychologist who screens both surrogates and couples for Surrogate Motherhood, Inc., in Maryland, has noted that couples fantasize quite a bit about the new women in their lives. "The wife goes through some natural feelings of inadequacy, that she is not a complete woman without children, and becomes afraid her husband will run off and find the perfect woman someplace. Those feelings were there before they came into the program, and they are always there to some degree. Yes, he has thought about it, but he has never done anything about it. Kind of healthy fantasy really. As long as you don't do it. It's a release."

Harrison also points out that people are usually defensive about their fantasies and do not want to talk about them. When asked, most couples deny even having those feelings.

Marilyn Smith says that her husband, never having lived with a pregnant woman, was so removed from the idea of children and childbearing that he did not even understand what was involved. She jokingly hinted that he thought babies came with the stork. "If he fantasized about the surrogate, I never had any clue whatsoever, and I would say he never did."

Anita Cody still feels envious of people who can get pregnant right away. "But I never felt any jealousy towards the surrogate, because she was doing it for me, really. I think she did it more for me than for Bart."

As soon as the contract between Dee and Carol and Peter Wright was signed in March, Dee sat down to write them a letter.

"It was a hard letter to write," says Dee. "How do you break the ice?"

She tried many times, but once she got going, "it turned out to be an easy letter to write. I just wanted them to know that I was committing myself to them to bring them the child that they wanted, and that I was doing it for them and not for me, that this was in fact their baby."

Dee and Carol exchanged letters about once a week.

"We got to know each other pretty well through letters," says Dee, and Carol agrees. "We felt pretty connected. Dee is a very open, warm person, and we immediately became good friends."

Carol adds, "Peter would tack on a little note at the end of the letter. He sort of wanted to be part of it, wanted to be involved, but the real emotional involvement was between Dee and me."

The pregnancy progressed normally and with the usual discomfort for Dee.

"There were probably some days when I was throwing up that I thought, 'Why couldn't it be her instead of me doing this?' but knowing that she had done everything possible to do this for herself, I never felt any resentment."

"I probably had a lot of needless concerns about the pregnancy," admits Carol. "Like once Dee wrote she had a bad cold, and I immediately worried about that, and she had a cat so I worried about toxoplasmosis. Once I wrote to ask her about her diet. I just wanted to know. I think it's just when you have been through the lengths we've been through to have a baby, you worry about everything."

There was really no need to.

Says Dee, "I was taking care of myself and the baby for those people. They had enough trust in me to do that for them, to play a part in their life, to bring them a child, and I tried as much as I could to make sure that I would give them a healthy baby."

Dee wrote to Carol faithfully and sent pictures of her stomach in profile.

"I always wanted Carol to feel as involved as possible, as pregnant as possible. I even told her to close her eyes and imagine real hard what I was feeling and she would feel it, too. In one of my letters I told her to put a volleyball under her shirt and bend over to try and shave her legs, because that's what I felt like when I was in the shower."

"We knew the baby was growing, and Dee gained weight beautifully—she only gained twenty-eight pounds," says Carol. "Dee was always, oh, she was always just the perfect surrogate. We could not have been any luckier."

Although the doctor found it unnecessary, Carol and Peter wanted amniocentesis to reassure themselves of the baby's health and Dee agreed. The results came back on Dee's birthday—"a very nice birthday present, that it was going to be a healthy baby." The test also told Carol and Peter that the balloons had not given them an accurate prediction of the sex of the baby. They were having a boy.

"It was a tremendous comfort to have the results," says Carol, and although they did not have any gender preference, "It was very important to know it was a boy. That was a real surge of reality, and we could start relating to him."

Where there is little contact between surrogate and couple, the future parents live in limbo.

When the Codys got news of their surrogate's pregnancy, they "were happy, but unsure," says Anita. "We only knew from the agency that she was pregnant. We got doctors' reports whenever she had a visit, but we didn't know for sure if there was a real baby. We got everything thirdhand and just hoped the whole things wasn't a hoax." Some months into the pregnancy they saw sonograms of the fetus, so "we knew there was a baby somewhere."

"There need to be tactics to make the adoptive mother involved," says Detroit psychiatrist Lawrence Turkow. "She seems to be the alien who has to look for a place to register."[7]

The Codys wanted to show the surrogate their appreciation, so for Christmas they sent the agency money to buy the surrogate a Christmas present—"I think they sent a bracelet," says Anita.

Some parents-to-be show their gratitude to the surrogate by showering them with presents.

Says a former assistant at Infertility Associates International, "Gifts come in; flowers are sent. One couple even sent their surrogate on vacation to Florida—the whole family. Some couples don't do anything. They don't want to know anything, because that's best for them."

But not getting any sign of appreciation is hard on the surrogate.

Says the former Infertility Associates International assistant, "There was one surrogate I sent letters to—not letters from the couple, but letters to her as if they were from the couple. She was just so elated when these letters came—'Oh, they are thinking of me.' Well, no letters ever came to the office. She needed that booster, and it didn't take any time for me to figure out something nice to say. She was elated, and when the baby was born everything was fine."

Fears About the Surrogate's Change of Mind

Well into Dee's pregnancy, the Baby M case came to the attention of the public. Here was a surrogate mother who refused to give up the baby girl, a pretty frightening precedent for people in a similar situation.

"I really didn't get worried," says Carol. "Dee wrote us and that was the key—'I know you are worried, but you don't have to be. This is your child.' And then she said one thing that clinched it for us—'You are as committed to take this baby as we are committed to giving it to you,' and we knew how committed we were!

She instilled the most incredible confidence in us. She was really very together about why she was doing it and her feelings about it.''

Nobody had ever heard of Baby M when Lorna Gallo got news of her surrogate's pregnancy. Although she was "pretty excited," she was even more scared.

"I was so afraid she was going to keep the baby. It was the hardest nine months of my life. I was petrified. I panicked bad. I wanted to call the whole thing off, because I felt I couldn't live like that.''

Linda corresponded with the surrogate, who sent reassuring letters—"She wrote me saying she was playing with her daughter, and she thought of us, and in a couple of months we would be playing with our baby.''

But the letters did not allay Linda's fears, and neither did therapy—"nothing did.''

Marilyn Smith applied a logical approach to her fears about the surrogate changing her mind.

"It wasn't something I really worried about. I tried to tell myself, 'If you can't do anything about it, don't worry about it until it happens.' I tried to keep a positive outlook on the whole thing.''

The hardest thing for Marilyn was answering people's queries.

"So many people would say, 'Do you really think she is going to give it up?' It creates a lot of negative questions in your mind when you're trying real hard to convince yourself that everything is going to work out. You have to defend yourself and also the surrogate and say, 'I feel real confident that she will.' One thing I will always be grateful to the surrogate for is her letters. Each time she would write and tell how the pregnancy was progressing, and she always referred to it as our baby—'Your baby is about so long now; your baby kicked today.' It was really a boost to us.''

The Moment of Truth

Dee had a problem-free pregnancy and a history of very short labor. Because it was winter and she had a forty-five-minute ride to the hospital, the doctor decided to induce labor. That gave Carol and Peter a chance to be at the hospital in Kansas for the birth and to meet Dee before the big moment.

"We met Dee on January seventh. It was very nerve-wracking.

We were very anxious,'' Carol remembers. "The Hagar Institute arranged for all of us to meet in the cafeteria of the hospital. We got there first and were wandering around the corridors. We were standing outside the ladies' room and saw Dee walk by. We knew immediately who she was. We sort of looked at each other— 'Now what do we do?' ''

They did nothing until Glenda from the Hagar Institute arrived and introduced them.

"I was real worried," says Dee. "What if they don't like me, what if they don't like the way I look?''

"Dee looked radiant and beautiful the day before giving birth. She just always looked so lovely in her pictures and in person as well," says Carol.

They hugged each other.

"That was just the most wonderful feeling," Dee remembers.

"Maybe it was all a little surreal, a little unreal," Carol muses. "I don't know what we talked about—probably the weather. We were in a state of shock—were we really going to have a baby tomorrow?''

"Well," Dee said. "Are you ready for the big day?''

And her son handed Carol and Peter a present she had bought and wrapped. It was a baby book. Denise had arranged for all the labor nurses to sign it and get the baby's footprints in it.

"It was just incredibly sweet and thoughtful," says Carol.

The doctor had set the induction for 8:00 the next morning, and Dee told them there was no need for them to come earlier than 9:00—"Take your time.''

Carol and Peter did not sleep a wink, and Carol cried off and on throughout the night.

When they got to the hospital the process had been started, and Dee was in control.

"Dee! The way she does everything! It was like she was showing up for a driver's test, she was so calm and collected," says Carol.

At 10:00 the doctor broke Dee's water in the labor room, but it did not speed up the delivery. So they all sat around and talked.

"Her husband was wonderful," says Carol. "He was telling us what was going on and what to expect. He really coached us because Dee was a pro and didn't need it, but we did. Dale said, 'I want you guys to relax.' ''

"He was just an incredible guy," says Peter.

After three hours of waiting, the doctor ordered Dee out of bed, so she walked around the hospital, pulling along the IV on little wheels.

"We have pictures of this parade of Dee, her husband, Glenda, Peter, and me walking around trying to get something going," Carol says, laughing.

Still nothing happened except that Carol and Peter chewed their fingernails, so at 2:30 the doctor was called and he gave Dee Pitocin intravenously, and then things happened. Labor really began.

"Dee was in such incredible control that it helped us handle it and stay in control."

The contractions quickly got intense and close together, and when Carol and Peter looked up, Dale was in his blue surgical gown and the nurses were opening the door to wheel Dee into the delivery room.

"Dee had asked us a couple of times if we wanted to be there for the birth, and we had never committed to it," admits Carol. "We are both a little squeamish and didn't know if it was going to be too much to handle. We didn't want to faint or get in anybody's way. We had told her that."

On leaving the room, a nurse threw them a couple of surgical gowns and said, "Okay, make up your minds, this is it."

They put on the gowns, and Peter had his camera around his neck.

The nurse said, "Why don't you go down the hall a bit. You can't see anything, but you can hear."

They went down the hall.

The nurse said, "Now that you're here, why don't you stand in the doorway?"

"We looked at each other and said, 'Let's do it.' It just felt right, and I think it was because of the way Dee handled the situation. I know it was," says Carol. "I felt an incredible gratitude to her through the entire process."

The nurse said, "Take a picture, why don't you?"

The doctor walked in five minutes before the delivery—"They always show up for the good part," said a nurse.

"Three pushes and the baby is out," the doctor predicted.

Dale was right by Dee, and Peter and Carol stood in the doorway "hanging on to each other" and "drifting into never-never land, not quite believing it yet."

"Sometimes I wish I could have had Carol right with me holding my hand and actually seeing everything," says Dee. "I'm glad they were there."

A host of nurses, all of whom knew a surrogate baby was being born, joined them. There were three pushes, Dee "let out a sort of yell at the very end," and then the doctor held up the baby— "It's a boy!"

"It was really incredible, so exciting, so wonderful," says Carol. "We were all crying, and hugging each other, all the nurses cried, too, and hugged us. It was incredible."

"Total tears," says Peter. "Everything over the last nine months was being brought to bear on this moment."

"I could hear them in the background," says Dee. "And that was the most wonderful thing to hear. I turned around and looked at them. They were embraced in each other, just crying, and what a wonderful thing it was to see. It was perfect."

The baby was wrapped in a blanket and put on a warming table, and Carol and Peter walked over to look at him.

A nurse said, "You can touch him. He's your son; you can hold him," and handed Carol the baby.

"Oh God, I just felt incredibly happy. It was the happiest moment of my life. He was such a beautiful little baby." Carol cannot think of the moment without crying again.

"When that baby was born, they forgot everything that was going on except for him. They took right over and that's exactly what I wanted them to do," says Dee.

The nurse then asked Dee if she wanted to hold the baby.

"No, not now," Dee said. "He is theirs; let them have this time."

Marilyn Smith's husband "thinks everything should run on schedule," so he expected their baby to arrive on its due date, February 22, 1986. The last week in January he decided that their house needed more insulation and tore down all the walls of their bedroom. Marilyn protested, "We don't have time to do this." But her husband was confident: "Oh no, we have plenty of time."

"On the eleventh of February, when they called from the hospital to tell us she was definitely in labor, my husband said, 'It's only the eleventh. Are you real sure?' "

Leaving insulation behind, Marilyn and her husband went to the hospital, but they did not want to witness the delivery of their baby. When the nurse called them in after the birth, Marilyn was "kind of scared." She had never met the surrogate before.

"She looked great, sitting up in bed. She had her hair combed and lipstick on," Marilyn says, full of admiration. "My husband thought she should be lying there half dead. They had a big rocking chair, and her husband very nicely pulled the rocking chair alongside the bed and says to me, 'Well, sit down,' and I did, and I didn't know what to expect. The surrogate kind of leaned forward, she handed the baby over and said, 'Here is your baby.' "

Marilyn was overwhelmed. "I was just about numb. For the first ten or fifteen minutes, I just could not take my eyes off that baby. It was like there was nobody else in the whole world. It was just like everybody else was pieces of furniture—I knew they were there, but I didn't pay one bit of attention, and I didn't care if they all got up and left. I stayed right in that chair.

"We wanted a boy," Marilyn confesses, "but we got a girl. I told my husband the day after she was born, 'I guess I was wrong. I must have wanted a girl the whole time.' He still wanted a boy, but he wouldn't give her up for anything in the world."

Lorna Gallo's surrogate delivered at home, and paramedics brought the baby to a nearby hospital.

"We got the baby when she was two hours old. I didn't cry," says Lorna. "I really thought I was going to cry, but I didn't. I was just real happy. The whole thing just felt so natural, like I was supposed to be doing it, that I didn't even think about it."

Lorna is immensely grateful to the surrogate. "My life was complete now because of a special person like herself."

The Codys' surrogate delivered at 3:00 in the morning. They were not allowed in the delivery room or to meet the surrogate, but they got the baby, Brian, "right after he was born."

Anita did not bond with the new baby immediately. She was still "shell-shocked" over the loss of the first baby. After two weeks, it suddenly hit her.

"I remember feeding him in the kitchen, and he was staring at me so intensely; it just made me melt. I can't explain the feeling. It was there and it wasn't there before. It was like he was part of me."

Anita admires the unknown woman who gave her a baby. "I wish I could do it for somebody. It is just a really wonderful thing to do, for a life is the most precious gift you can give. I wish I could walk up and shake her hand."

The delivery of Carmen and Ted Dubois's first baby was traumatic. The surrogate mother almost bled to death.

"It was quite emotional, and I stayed up there for three solid weeks," says Carmen. It was a difficult situation because the hospital did not know the child was a surrogate baby, and the surrogate's husband was afraid the hospital would get wind of it, so "it was not a happy situation, because I could not see her and I could not see the baby. We didn't know from day to day, half the time, what was going on. I didn't know if I was going to lose the baby altogether." The surrogate mother wanted Carmen to be there, but her husband was so upset "that he wasn't thinking clearly,'' and he is still so distraught that Carmen cannot contact the woman she had grown close to. But Carmen got her baby, and the surrogate mother recovered. Their second baby arrived safely a few months later.

Peter and Carol spent three days at the hospital with Dee. They had a small room where they "lived" from 7:00 in the morning until 10:30 at night.

Carol and Peter were taking care of the baby, but "it didn't seem real at all—it did seem like playing house," Carol says. "We had been waiting forever for this."

Dee would wander in and they would visit Dee's room between feeding and changing the baby.

"It was like they had had a baby and we had had a baby the same time in the same hospital—the same baby, of course. A lot of denial going on, I'm sure," says Carol, "but it was remarkable how comfortable it was."

The day after Matthew was born, Carol was sitting with him in the rocking chair when Dee came for a visit. Dee commented upon how contented Carol looked and said she hoped the baby would be as good at home as he was in the hospital. Carol asked Dee if she would like to hold the baby.

"I guess so," Dee answered, and sat down in the rocking chair with the baby.

Matthew started to fuss, and Dee said, "Oh no. Look, he's not happy. He knows I'm not the mother." And she handed him right back to Carol.

"Dee always had such respect for our feelings throughout this whole thing," says Carol with gratitude. "She was absolutely phenomenal."

All of them—Carol, Peter, Dee, and Dale—began to realize that it would be hard to say goodbye to each other. They had developed a relationship "that wasn't in anybody's dictionary."

Toward the end of the hospital stay Carol wandered into Dee's room.

"I went into her room just to shoot the breeze, and I started weeping, just crying, and at that point I said, 'Dee, do you have any idea what you have done for us?' "

"No, I really can't imagine what you have been through," Dee said, "but I'm just glad that you are happy."

"And we just stood there crying and hugging each other for what seemed like an eternity."

"It was harder to leave Carol and Peter than the baby," Dee says. "I had attached myself more to them than to the baby. This was not a child conceived from my love and my husband's love, but their love; and to see them with their baby was wonderful. I had no second thought about relinquishing at all.''

Neither did Dale. "I had no feelings for the baby at all," he insists.

There were many goodbyes. At the official one, Carol and Peter gave Dee a necklace with little diamonds in it, and Dale, for distinguished service during the delivery, received a T-shirt proclaiming, "I'm the coach." And the tears flowed again.

Dee and Dale left the hospital first. As they were checking out right across from Carol and Peter's room, there was time for one last quick goodbye.

"This was going to be the low-key goodbye, the we-don't-have-to-cry-because-we-already-cried goodbye, the easy one, but we cried all over again," Peter admits.

"It takes a big bang for my husband to drop a tear," says Dee, "but he sure cried, too."

Carol and Peter watched Dee and Dale go through the doors. They they looked at each other and said, "There go two incredible people."

"When we got out in the parking lot, we sat in the car for a minute, and they came to the window and were waving at us," says Dee. "And that was the last we saw of them. But to this day I feel they are the best friends in the world, that they would always be there for me. I'm glad we did it."

"It was their big chance to have a family," says Dale.

"We feel blessed," say Carol and Peter.

Little Matthew's baby book starts with pictures of all four of them in the delivery room.

Adjusting to the Baby

In fiction, the stories would stop with the happy parents taking home their child, but this is real life, and new parents have to learn to adjust their lives to a new baby that has been endowed with dreamlike perfection and then turns out to be a wailing nuisance from time to time.

Constance Shapiro, who counsels infertile couples, warns all such new parents not to expect too much. "Infertile people who become parents must be watchful of the tendency to expect perfection of their children, to expect of their children confirmation of their expectations as parents."

It would not be odd to find there was a letdown for the parents after nine months of almost unbearable expectation.

Dee's husband, Dale, who is raising his own "two little monsters," thinks that perhaps the novelty has worn off a bit for Carol and Peter: "They were very excited, but I think as the months wore on, their letters have changed to some extent—the routine and everything. It is a lot of work, and I don't think they realized it is a lot of work. They had no idea before they got into it, and they got their hands full and their feet wet. You know, the newness wears off. Reality sets in."

Carol, though, says that "the thrill hasn't worn off. In the beginning friends would call us and say, 'You will get through this early stage; it gets better.' We would sort of look at each other and say, 'We are enjoying every minute of this.' "

Carol realizes that the circumstances of Matthew's birth may well cause some problems later on. "I'm not saying it's not going to have its tough moments, but the one thing we always felt, when he gets older he will never have one minute where he thinks he was an unwanted child." She feels he has that advantage over an adopted child. "To me that is the plus in all of this because it *is* weird, it is unusual. Sure, I wish I never had had to do it. I wish I were the mother."

For Marilyn Smith's husband, every stage seems a mystery. Says Marilyn, "The first few months, he was kind of afraid of her. He used to say, 'When is the baby going to do something? She just lays there.' Now, fifteen months later, he says, 'Doesn't that kid ever shut up, ever sit down quietly?' "

Lorna Gallo is the proud mother. Annie, now fifteen months old, does "all the things that babies are supposed to do," but "of course, she's doing more. She loves being a parrot; everything you say, she repeats it. She is into everything. She is a real good baby, though, a real good baby."

Carmen Dubois had quite a bit of adjustment to do. After the babies, born three months apart, came home, "there were still some emotions that surfaced, because my husband left me with absolutely no help. It was enough that I had to accept children that didn't belong to me, but I also had to take care of the children that didn't belong to me."

Although Carmen realized that "the babies had absolutely nothing to do with it," it still took her a good year to really accept them.

There she was at home with two children, having left her job as a lab assistant, struggling with her pent-up emotions—"I'm some forty years old. What am I doing? These aren't my children. I don't love them. How can I accept it?"

She went through the motions of mothering. "I handled them like a robot. You know what you're supposed to do—I fed them, I changed them, I rocked them—but your feelings . . ." In retrospect though, says Carmen, "It really wasn't all that bad. Having two made it a lot easier on me, and there wasn't any problem."

The two girls are almost four years old now, and they are happily going to nursery school, where everybody knows about the circumstances of their birth, "simply because there is only a three-and-a-half-month difference" between them. The girls get along "beautifully."

"I think having two has helped tremendously—far better than having just one," Carmen feels.

Carmen is going to tell them about their biological mothers when they are a little older. "Right now they are very happy, well-adjusted children. The impact will come when they are, oh, around eight or nine years old."

She is not expecting big problems.

"We made it a point to choose highly intelligent surrogates. We're kind of banking on the fact that with that background, they will grow up to be very sensitive, sincere children. And as it stands now, they have shown to be exactly what we're looking for. There are no disappointments whatsoever."

Carmen had agreed to have surrogate children mainly to please her husband, "but that has changed." The feeling of resentment "is gone completely," she says. "These two are just something else!"

The Adoption Hitch

Surrogate babies are the children of the surrogate and the man who provided the sperm. The infertile wife, for whose benefit these babies are usually created, has no biological connection or legal claim to them at all. Surrogate mothers have to relinquish their rights to the child, and the infertile wife, to make the child legally hers, has to adopt it.

Even if the surrogate gives up the child immediately, adoption is not always straightforward. In some states the child of a woman who has been artificially inseminated automatically becomes the child of the woman's husband. His name and not the donor's appears on the birth certificate, thus depriving the biological father of parental rights. These laws were enacted to avoid the stigma of illegitimacy for children conceived by donor sperm, but they complicate surrogate adoptions. The way to get around that problem is for the husband of the surrogate mother to sign a form indicating that he does not consent to his wife's artificial insemination, leaving the sperm donor free to claim the child.

The surrogate mother, of course, has the right not to sign the release papers and fight for custody, as happened in the Baby M case. Although in that case the biological father was eventually awarded custody, there is no guarantee of the same outcome if another biological mother should change her mind. Most surrogates do sign the release papers immediately so that the couple can begin adoption procedures.

Marilyn Smith and her husband retained a lawyer to help them with the formalities, but they were still in for a surprise. After the surrogate had signed the release papers and Marilyn wanted to take the baby home, the nurses said, "Oh no, you're not taking her." The baby had to stay in the hospital. It turned out that Marilyn needed a temporary custody order.

"Nobody had told us that was necessary, so we had to run and track down the judge and get him—against his better judgment—to sign the order. It was very difficult."

That was only the first hurdle. When it came to the adoption proceedings, they got a judge who was not in favor of surrogacy. Luckily Marilyn's attorney knew the judge "quite well," so she took the judge aside and told him, "Look, this is a court case. You cannot let your personal feelings enter into it."

The judge nevertheless balked.

"He made us go through another home study because he didn't know the Hagar Institute from a hole in the wall," says Marilyn, "and he wasn't going to take what they had written on a piece of paper as anything he could trust."

Marilyn got nervous, wondering what was going to happen. She went through the court-mandated home study to get certified as a good parent for the second time. "After it was all over, I was kind of glad," she says, "because they came up with a good report. It seemed to them that the Hagar Institute had done a very thorough job."

Peter and Carol knew from the beginning that the adoption was going to be complicated. Their home state, Massachusetts, does not allow privately arranged adoptions, and neither does Missouri, Dee's home state, so they adopted in Kansas. Dee signed the relinquishment papers twenty-four hours after Matthew was born, so that was no problem, but the judge who had been finalizing adoptions in cases where both the surrogate and the adoptive mother were from out of state decided a month before the baby was born "that she couldn't do it any more; she really didn't have jurisdiction." Peter and Carol got themselves a Massachusetts lawyer and had another home study.

They left the hospital on a Sunday and went to stay with friends until the court allowed them to go home. Suddenly they were without the hospital support staff.

"It was sheer terror," Carol remembers, "because we didn't have the nurses there to brief us. We didn't sleep one second. It was scary."

The next morning they bundled up the baby and took him out in freezing weather to drive an hour and a half to Topeka for a five-minute court session. Their lawyer had done her homework, so "the judge just wanted to see the baby and meet us. She signed the papers and that was it."

But they could not go home.

"We had to hang around for these official types to get around to signing the interstate compact," Carol explains. "It is an agreement between states saying that if a baby is leaving one state and being accepted into another, each state will comply with the regulations drawn up between them."

That came through the following Wednesday, and they could finally go home.

The plane trip to Massachusetts "was sort of fun," says Carol. "Everybody came up and said, 'What a beautiful baby. How old is he?' "

People told Carol, "Gee, you look wonderful!"

"Thanks," she said. "I feel wonderful!"

Friends and relatives were waiting at the airport with flowers and a limousine, and the whole arrival was captured on videotape.

Thirty days later the adoption became final, and Dee sent them a bouquet of balloons in celebration.

Carol and Dee still correspond, and Carol carries one of Dee's letters with her at all times.

7

The Women Who Serve as Surrogates

THE RECEPTIONIST CALLS JANET REID, TWENTY-FIVE, OVER THE
office phone, and a minute later she appears in the lobby of a
Washington, D.C., law firm where she works as a legal secretary.
She has pretty shoulder-length red hair and her face is very dis-
creetly made up. She is wearing a crisp blue dress with a lowered
waistline that makes her look pregnant. Another one? Janet gave
birth to a surrogate baby in September 1986.

In the elevator down, without any prompting, she pats her stomach and says, "This one is for me."

Sitting at a small table in the restaurant she scans the menu for
something filling and nutritious and orders an omelet.

"During my first pregnancy I gained sixty pounds," she says. It
is hard to believe; she does not look a bit overweight and her
pregnancy hardly shows. "I lost fifty pounds in three months, but
then I got pregnant again before I lost the last ten."

Surrogates are often thought of as odd and different from the
standard idea of a woman, and as if to confirm that view of
surrogate mothers, Janet says, "I'm not the normal person. I do
things that are very outlandish, very outspoken, and things that are
a bit risky."

Risky indeed. The Baby M case showed the world that surrogate motherhood is strewn with emotional dangers and thorny legal and moral questions. Several European countries where surrogate motherhood is virtually unknown are considering legislation to ban the practice before it takes hold. England has already outlawed surrogacy agencies. So why would anybody want to get into it?

"To be quite frank, money is the main drive. It is a way to earn money. You don't have to work a second job, it's your own time, it doesn't affect you—of course it affects you, but it doesn't affect you like a second job, where you're exhausted when you come home and you have to get there every day. I thought it was a nice way to help me and help someone else at the same time. You do something to get yourself out of a hole and something to complete someone else's life. It's double payback for me. It was well worth it. At that point I didn't feel I had accomplished anything, and this gave me a feeling of self worth that I could never do on my own."

She does not seem to be suffering from any lack of self-esteem. Quite the contrary. She carries herself with a great deal of self-assurance and balance. But one wonders if maybe there are troubling details in her past. Psychiatrist Philip Parker at Wayne State University School of Medicine studied over 200 surrogate mothers and found that about one-third of them had previously voluntarily aborted or given up a child for adoption and saw surrogate motherhood as a way to atone for a deed they now regretted.

No, Janet never had—nor would ever have—an abortion, and she never gave a child up for adoption. Her childhood, though, was not a Norman Rockwell idyll. Her parents divorced when she was very young, and although she has some contact with her father, they are not close. She lived with her mother, two sisters, and a brother until age eleven, when her mother, a manic depressive, went to a mental institution that she has been in and out of ever since. Janet's grandparents cared for her until she was seventeen, when she struck out on her own.

"I'm a very cut-and-dried person. That's what the psychologist who screened me said: 'You deal with your feelings—you put them away in the attic and you never touch them again.' That's the best way for my personality. I mean, if the door comes open and I have a problem to solve, fine, I'll deal with it, but I don't open the door by myself and say, 'Oh, let's deal with one.' I've always been that way."

Janet never told her mother about her decision to become a surrogate mother, and she also kept her grandparents in the dark.

"They are of the generation where they just couldn't fathom

why I would have a child, being single, and ruin my life, as they would say—'Now you'll never get married.' ''

The rest of the family knew.

"I think my father was proud of me, once he got used to the idea. My sister, who has a daughter, couldn't believe I was going to do it. She said, 'Janet, there is no way, once the baby starts moving in your stomach, you're going to be able to handle it.' My other sister, who had a baby at eighteen and gave it up for adoption, she understood what I would be facing, and it was much harder for her because she was in love with someone and it was their child. She was always backing me up. My brother really didn't care what I did. To me it felt like a science project.''

Janet was brought up Catholic and the church is dead-set against the practice of surrogacy, but Janet was not concerned.

"I know the Catholic church denounces surrogate parenting and everything else. They denounce everything that moves. I think it is foolish.''

In spite of conflicting advice and church disapproval, Janet was convinced she could handle surrogate motherhood.

"I'm sentimental, but I also have a stiff backbone, and once I set my standards, I follow through. If I have problems, I'll solve the problems, get back on track.''

So she called a local sperm bank and asked for references to surrogate agencies. There were two in her area. One rejected her right away because she had not proven her fertility by a previous pregnancy, but the other one accepted her, provided her physical examination and psychological testing turned out okay. They did, and she signed a contract promising her $10,000, to be held in escrow until the baby was born. After three rounds of artificial insemination with an unknown man's sperm, she became pregnant.

"I really didn't care whether my family or the people at work got upset, because I'm just that type of person. I do what makes me happy, and if people don't like it, they don't have to stand around me. In the office, people were reserved; they didn't want to talk to me. They were afraid I would get too involved, so they were afraid to discuss it with me. I could always talk about it—it was my life for a whole year. I mean, the baby's moving—it's a thrill, it's exciting, how can you ignore it? They would always say, 'That's nice,' and go on with their lunch. They didn't want to talk about it. It made them nervous.

"People who didn't know *would* bring it up—'Oh, you're pregnant!', and would ask me if I had named the baby or gotten the room ready. If I was in a bad mood, I would say, 'Yeah, yea, I've named it; it's ready.' In a good mood, I would chitchat and say, 'Oh, it isn't mine; it's a surrogate baby,' and I loved watching their faces. Suddenly there is surprise and then they would try to mask it.

"Some people didn't understand what *surrogate* meant. I could see them just dying to get to a dictionary to look it up—*surrogate, surrogate, surrogate*. I still went to my social spots after hockey games, and people at the bars were thrilled with it. They had a blast. I loved it. I am very much a ham. People were in awe of what I could do. I was all of a sudden superwoman."

The agency that arranged Janet's surrogate deal, Surrogate Motherhood, Inc., does not allow any contact between the contracting couple and the surrogate mother. The couple saw a picture of Janet and were given some information on her background, medical and social, but they do not know her name, nor she theirs. They never meet. Only secondhand contact is possible, through the director of the agency.

"Sharon [Whiteley, the director] would relate little snippets to me about how excited the couple was, and she would tell the couple about my little escapades while I was pregnant, like when I got sick on the train. I wanted the wife to experience her pregnancy—I do not think of it as my pregnancy—and she really appreciated knowing each step that I went through: when the baby started to move or little things that he would do. The adoptive mother recently said to the director that every time she looks at the baby, she thinks of me and thanks God I was born. They are very sweet and caring."

Janet delivered a healthy baby boy in September 1986, and her aunt, with whom she had taken Lamaze classes, was her coach.

"I held him when he was born, after they had cleaned him all up and the nurse was ready to hightail it out of the room, because they knew it was a surrogate baby. I said, 'Whoa,' and grabbed her skirt. 'Get back here!' And she looks at the doctor, and he is like, 'Okay, it's her baby,' and I held him. He was crying, and my aunt was crying profusely. Holding him it really felt like someone had gone to the nursery, taken somebody's child out of a basket, and handed it to me. I couldn't believe that that was from me. I guess, having a first child, I had never experienced how awesome it is to give birth to a child. He looked huge to me; I just couldn't believe he came out of me. Of course, I felt like it.

"The day after I had the baby, the pediatrician came in and checked him out and said, 'The baby is fine. He can be released.'

I signed the release papers. That was it; he was gone the next day. It was that quick."

Anonymity was maintained throughout. The parents and the director of the agency were waiting outside the hospital to receive the baby.

"My friend Cathy walked with the nurse who carried the baby— she wouldn't even let Cathy carry the baby out of the hospital. The director was waiting there with the car seat, and the nurse put the baby in the seat—no one could touch him—and made sure that everything was okay and secure. The director then took the baby around—my friend couldn't go with her, because she didn't want a friend to see who the couple is. The baby was brought around and the couple put the car seat in their car and, poof, they had a son."

Janet is in favor of keeping surrogate arrangements anonymous, but anonymity can go too far. Janet objects to the cloak and dagger approach.

"It just makes it seem so awful. Something like this makes people think of black market babies, because you have to have these clandestine meetings in the bushes. People are just so paranoid, and they make it seem worse than it is."

Baby selling is of course the critical term in discussions about surrogate parenting. Are surrogates selling babies or services?

"I didn't have any feelings that it's immoral," says Janet. "I could never in my life sell a baby for ten thousand dollars. There is no price on human life and happiness. The fee was for my suffering. Each one of my stretch marks is a thousand dollars. That's how I look at it.

"I made a down payment on a townhouse with the money and also cleared up a lot of my bills. It really felt wonderful carrying all that money to the bank and writing out those checks."

But what about giving up the baby? It must be hard.

Not for Janet. She was never attached to the fetus, and the fact that she and the couple had nothing to do with each other helped prevent any involvement with the baby, she thinks.

"I went through postpartum depression, but what was missing was the entity in my stomach, not the actual baby, my flesh and blood baby. I think about him now and then, and how the couple must be feeling, but I don't think of him in a sad way. It doesn't bother me. It doesn't keep me up nights. I don't cry about it. I don't mind the couple knowing who I am; they don't have to worry about me. If they popped in and said, 'Look, here's your son,' I would go, 'Oh, he's very cute.' That's about the only feeling I would get. I mean, he's gotten the best deal as far as deals go.''

If Janet's grandparents were kept in the dark about the surrogate baby because they couldn't fathom what she was doing, they may also have a hard time with the one on the way. It is an accidental pregnancy that happened the first time she had sex after delivering the surrogate baby—about three months after. The father ran for the hills. She is going through with the pregnancy.

"Once again you deal with it. That's my whole thing in life. Things come up and you deal with them, and they go away, more or less. This one won't go away for a long time. At first I thought, 'Am I ready for this?' I have never thought of single parenthood in my life. But now that the baby is moving—I'm in the sixth month now—it gets exciting. I start thinking about it more, and start thinking about the nursery. I just never could picture myself as the maternal type—it's coming out of its own accord. But yet, when I was a surrogate, I wouldn't even let the feelings begin to seed, I wouldn't put the seed in the soil, but now that I allow myself to drop it, it just, pfsh, it's gone. People are laughing hearing me go off on it, when they know I was so reserved and never thought a thing about it while I was pregnant as a surrogate. It's just amazing the difference.''

Janet is an all-American girl—healthy, intelligent, independent. She exhibits good time-honored American values: smarts, enterprise, courage, and no fear of new frontiers. And like a good American capitalist, she knows the value of money.

Janet is just one of the many hundreds of women who have volunteered their reproductive services to surrogate agencies, which link them up with infertile couples.

Becoming a Surrogate

Before a candidate is accepted into a surrogate program, she is tested. Surrogate agencies differ in their requirements and procedures, but all of them insist on a medical examination and a psychological evaluation to test their physical and emotional health.

The medical tests are fairly routine but comprehensive.

"They test your heart, take your blood pressure, your temperature, a pap test, and check for venereal disease,'' says Joan Field, a surrogate in Clovis, California. "And they do blood work, a whole bunch of tests. I can't even begin to remember, but a lot—anything that could interfere with pregnancy. It is a routine thing.''

In the psychological exam, Joan answered 560 true/false questions on the Minnesota Multiphasic Personality Index (MMPI), a test that reveals personality disorders. She also had a long interview and an I.Q. test.

Kandy Harris, twenty-five, who lives with her husband, Chris, a pizza parlor manager, and their three-year-old daughter in Kansas City, found the screening done by the Hagar Institute "quite rigorous."

"They wanted references, they did a home study. When I first called them, it was, 'Why do you want to do this.' . . . They had me go through a psychologist who did an MMPI, and I.Q. test, and a personal interview."

A surrogate has to be in good health to be accepted, but she also has to show a strong psychological profile. Being a surrogate puts her in an unusual emotional situation, especially at the time when she relinquishes the child. Surrogacy is still such a new area for psychologists that they are still not sure what it takes to be a good surrogate.

Dennis Harrison, a forensic psychologist who screens surrogate candidates for Surrogate Motherhood, Inc., in Maryland, does not look for special characteristics in a surrogate.

"Primarily you try to rule out some things, rule out people who have emotional problems," he says. "To look at it from the positive end, we want somebody who has got the ability to communicate, someone who has got the ability to be flexible emotionally, to deal with situations—somebody who isn't too rigid."

Psychologist Philip Parker, who screens surrogates for Noel Keane's Michigan office, has said, "I wouldn't know what a good surrogate is. For all we know, the more disturbed she is the better."[1] But most people involved in the selection of candidates tend to take a more conventional approach.

Dr. Joan Einwohner, a psychologist who acts as consultant for Keane's Infertility Institute in New York City, tries to cut down on the margin of error.

"I tend to reject extremes. This is all such a brand-new field. You really don't know who will be a good surrogate and who won't, who won't be able to carry it through without negative consequences to themselves. I choose a conservative point of view. I reject eighteen to twenty percent of the surrogates I see."

Matthew Meyers, the lawyer for Surrogate Motherhood, Inc., is equally leery of extremes.

"One of the things we are looking for in a surrogate is a stable person who is not going to sway with the wind under pressure. Part of what we are looking to screen out is extreme emotions and reactions on any end of the spectrum, because those people are much harder to predict in a crisis."

To keep the surrogates on a steady course, many agencies offer them psychological counseling throughout the pregnancy and a few months after the delivery.

If a surrogate passes the psychological and medical tests, she is eventually linked up with an infertile couple. In some cases the surrogates meet with the couple for whom they will bear children. In other cases, the couples are little more than a brief description on a piece of paper given to the surrogates by the agency.

Some surrogates have specific requirements for the couple for whom they will work. One early Keane surrogate, a midwife from Texas with one son, wanted no money for carrying a child to be given up but had a ten-point list of demands.

1. The child will be born at home, with the supervision of midwives.
2. The adoptive mother *must* be present for the birth.
3. If at all possible, the adoptive father and any siblings should be present.
4. The adoptive parents must be willing to have the child breast-fed for three to five days in order for the child to receive the benefit of my calostrum.
5. The child is at no time to be placed in a foster home during adoption proceedings.
6. The adoptive parents pay any medical expenses involving miscarriage or prematurity.
7. The adoptive parents demonstrate financial and emotional security and a willingness to educate themselves on all aspects of childrearing.
8. The adoptive parents be personally involved during the prenatal period, they be willing to exchange feelings with me, and they be honest with friends and relatives about what they are doing. The parents should feel joy and antici-pation, not guilt or doubt.
9. The mother can afford to spend at least three months at home with her baby.
10. That the parents have no wish to "forget" me after the birth. They must realize I can never forget what I've done for them.[2]

"The idea that needs to be more prominent," says Donna Regan, twenty-four, a Noel Keane surrogate married to a machine operator, "is that surrogates who go in don't have to work with a couple. We have as much choice as the couple does. If you don't feel comfortable with a certain couple, you certainly don't want to carry a child for them."

"One thing that was very important to me," says Donna, "was how are they going to raise these children? Are they going to raise them with the same amount of love and care I would want children raised with?"

Some agencies do not allow the surrogate to impose demands on a couple. The surrogate's main options lie in picking and choosing the parents from the files forwarded to her by the agency.

Kandy, though, had a whole string of requirements.

First of all, she did not want to be related to the child she was going to give birth to. She was willing to carry the child but not to donate an egg. Kandy wanted to be an *in vitro* surrogate. Luckily, when she signed up with the Hagar Institute, medical science had progressed so far that it was possible to extract one or more eggs from a woman, fertilize the eggs in a petri dish, and implant the resulting embryo in the womb of a surrogate. This method allows a woman with no uterus but with functioning ovaries to have her own genetic child carried to term by a surrogate. However, the success rate of *in vitro* fertilization is not very high when involving just one woman; with two women participating in the creation of a child, it becomes even more complicated. Few couples who have already gone through years of infertility treatments have the emotional stamina to endure any more failures. And few couples can afford to pay the bills for *in vitro* fertilization on top of fees to the surrogate and the agency. However, even though it took a long time, Kandy was linked up with a couple and became the second woman in the United States to give birth to a child she was genetically unrelated to.

But Kandy had other demands. She wanted the child to "have the option of going to college." She did not want the couple to be smokers, and she would not have an abortion.

She straightened it out with her couple. "We agreed that if it was Down's syndrome or something like that, we would not abort. If it was something where the child would be in pain and an abortion was not just for the convenience of the parents, that would be different."

Surrogates and the Medical Establishment

Once the surrogate has agreed to work with a couple, artificial inseminations start.

Lisa Waters, thirty-two, a married college graduate with two children of her own, came from Wisconsin to Washington for her inseminations.

"The insemination was no big deal," she says. "Anybody who has had a pelvic examination has gone through that."

Insemination is a simple, painless procedure that takes place in a doctor's office.

"We treat the surrogate like we would any other patient," says Dr. Jeffrey Levitt, did one of Lisa's inseminations. "If it is their first time, they might be a little nervous, but I give them a *People* magazine. I talk to them, I show them all the instruments and tables while they are still completely dressed, and then we sit down and do it."

However, when Lisa got home to Wisconsin, she went for prenatal care to the doctor whom she had gone to "for years and years and years" and who had brought her through her previous pregnancies. But, she admits, "he didn't like the idea at all."

"Just the look in his eyes and the way his demeanor changed when I told him what I was doing told me that."

She found herself another doctor who was not personally opposed to surrogacy.

Another surrogate went to a hospital in the Washington, D.C., area to ask if they would deliver the baby, and the answer was, "We certainly would not."

Even if a hospital does accept surrogates as patients, the staff may show its displeasure. One surrogate was quizzed by a nurse who wheeled her to her room after an exhausting labor and delivery. "I know it is a bad time to ask," the nurse said, "but why did you decide to give up your baby for money?"[3]

The medical establishment may be uncomfortable with surrogacy, but that is no longer much of a stumbling block. In the early days, most physicians, fearing malpractice suits, refused even to inseminate surrogates. The very first surrogate trio—an infertile couple, George and Debbie, and their friend Sue, a virgin who had offered to have a baby for them—contacted several doctors in Michigan only to be turned down. They then decided to take the matter of life into their own hands. Debbie went to the drugstore and bought a couple of syringes, and with the help of the *Reader's Digest Family Health Guide*, which contains a precise description of how artificial insemination is done, Debbie filled the syringe with George's sperm after a session of interrupted lovemaking and proceeded to inseminate Sue. They hit the jackpot on the first try.

After the baby was born, Debbie and George ran into trouble with the medical establishment again. At the adoption proceedings in court, everything went smoothly until the doctor observed to Debbie, "Do you know you were practicing medicine without a license?"

Debbie shot back, "Now, wait a minute, doctor. You know as well as I do that we have approached several doctors, including yourself, to perform these inseminations and the doctors simply don't want to get involved. The next case I have I am going to ask you to do the artificial insemination, so we won't have laymen practicing medicine without a license."[4]

And that was the end of that.

Few doctors achieve the desired result as quickly as Debbie. Even though surrogates keep temperature charts to pinpoint the time of ovulation, the insemination rarely takes the first time. If too many cycles go by without a pregnancy, Dr. Jeffrey Levitt puts the surrogates on Clomid, which stimulates ovulation.

"Yes, we get them ovulating," he says. "I don't give Clomid because of pressure, but a lot of surrogates are not from this state. They will come in and the husbands will fly in, so you may have to modify things. Suppose somebody has an irregular cycle. Well, you've got to make them regular, so there are things you do. If I speed up things, it's because I feel it's ethically acceptable."

Inseminations are medically simple and painless, but for the newest kinds of stand-in mothers, *in vitro* surrogates, the procedure is not a simple routine. An *in vitro* surrogate does not get sperm injected into her vagina. She has an embryo transferred directly into her uterus.

Kandy remembers the procedure all too well. "They have this catheter, and they run it up through the vagina and the cervix into the uterus," she explains. "That hurts a lot, because to get through the cervix, they use these long scissors to hold it open. It was just like being in labor."

Kandy went through the embryo transfer three times before achieving pregnancy.

The Surrogate's Husband

Once a surrogate conceives, she not only has physical changes to contend with, she also has to be prepared for the reactions of people around her, not least her husband, if she has one.

Most husbands need a little persuading before agreeing with their wives that getting into surrogacy is a good idea.

Says Lisa Waters, "My husband's initial reaction wasn't all that positive. He thought I had gone off the deep end, but as time went on and he saw how committed I was to this idea, and as we got involved in the program, he became far more accepting. In the end he was just as enthusiastic as I was about it."

Kandy Harris's husband, Chris, was hesitant in the beginning.

"I initially remember thinking it was best for us to have the children we might want first, in case there were complications," Chris says. "I hesitated at first, but we talk out things pretty well most of the time. I feel Kandy is a smart person, so I trust her judgment. I'm pretty open as far as letting people do what they want to do, if they feel they should do it."

Some agencies put the surrogate husbands through a psychological test as well to make sure there are not hidden antagonisms toward the wife's decision. If the husband is not supportive, the surrogate is rejected.

Says Hilary Hanafin, a psychologist at the Center for Surrogate Parenting in Los Angeles, "With the husbands there is a lot of self-selection. If they don't approve of the idea, I usually don't see the wife. The husbands that make the interview tend to be genuinely supportive and empathetic.

"There are usually two types of husbands. One is the type that basically says, 'I love my wife; I think she can do this and I will support her, not because it is important to me but because it is something she wants to do.' The other type is one who has a lot more emotional motivation and has a lot of sympathy for a couple without a child, one who talks about how wonderful being a dad is."

The husband has to make sacrifices. When signing a contract, the surrogates promise to abstain from sex from approximately two weeks before the first insemination attempt until pregnancy is achieved, and that can be many months.

Regular vaginal sex before pregnancy would have constituted a breach of contract in Lisa Waters' case and was "punishable" by a $25,000 penalty. It took over four months for her to conceive, but luckily there are more ways between heaven and earth to have sex than missionaries have dreamed of, so for Lisa and her husband, Don, "it wasn't difficult. We didn't even have to struggle over that one." A couple of times when Don began to get careless, Lisa would say, "Hey, buddy, it's twenty-five thousand dollars," and he would back right off.

Kandy had to abstain from vaginal sex for no less than ten months until the embryo implant took. She did not feel it was a problem, and neither did her husband.

"I wouldn't say it was hard," says Chris, "but I don't feel real comfortable talking about it."

For Barbara Delsanto's husband, abstention was too difficult.

"He said, 'That's going to be too much of a problem for me, and it was. Even though he is only a few years younger than I, I always call my husband a sexpot. He loves me a lot, he wants to show me all the time. We did it," Barbara confesses. "We didn't do it while I was ovulating, but we didn't go along with that bull. After the baby was born and they were going through the paternity tests, I was super nervous."

The tests showed that no "accidents" had happened in this case, but there has been at least one case where paternity was disputed by the sperm donor.

In 1983 Alexander Malahoff, for whom Noel Keane had arranged a surrogate contract, refused to accept the baby born to surrogate mother, Judy Stiver, the wife of Ray Stiver, a bus driver in Michigan. The baby boy was sickly, suffered from micro-encephaly—he was born with an abnormally small brain—and was in all likelihood retarded. This was not what Mr. Malahoff, an accountant, had bargained for, and he was convinced that he could not have fathered the defective child. Blood tests were ordered to establish paternity, and the case hit the press in a big way. Phil Donahue persuaded both Mr. Malahoff and the Stivers to go on his television show while they waited for the results of the test. When it was announced on the air that Mr. Malahoff couldn't possibly be the father, he looked triumphant and the Stivers naturally pained. How was it possible? It turned out that Mrs. Stiver had been impregnated by her husband the day before she was artificially inseminated with Mr. Malahoff's sperm. It also turned out that microencephaly ran in Ray Stiver's family and that he had previously fathered a child suffering from the same condition.

But that is not the end of the story. Mr. Malahoff sued Judy Stiver for $50 million, charging breach of contract, the Stivers in turn sued Malahoff for invasion of privacy, and both sued Noel Keane and four doctors. The baby stayed with the Stivers.

Reactions of the Surrogate's "Own" Children

News of pregnancy is happy news. For the future parents it is the beginning of the fulfillment of their dream, and for the surrogates it means that they can resume a somewhat more normal routine for a while—no monthly traveling to doctors' offices for inseminations and no abstention from sex. They can get on "with the job."

Surrogate Katie Abrams, twenty-nine, was "ecstatic." Katie and her husband, a district sales manager for a retail firm in North Carolina, have three children of their own, and they all arrived a little sooner than expected. She got pregnant on her honeymoon, and the two younger children also had their own ideas of when to be born. She started artificial insemination in February 1986 and got pregnant in March.

"I was more ecstatic at being pregnant with their child than with my own," she says. "That sounds crazy, but I had never tried to get pregnant, and I knew how long these people had tried, seven years. I cried. I knew how much a baby meant to these people."

Surrogates are usually advised to explain their unusual decision to their own children before inseminations start, but if they have not, there is no skirting the issue once the pregnancy shows.

Lisa Waters' three-year-old son was amazed to see her stomach grow so big that he could not sit on her lap; her four-year-old son was "cool" about it.

"We told them from the day I decided to get involved in it that Mommy was going to have a baby, but it wasn't ours, but for another mom and dad who can't have any. They accepted that. Once they get old enough to realize that not everybody's mom does this, they will have more questions, but we have just answered whatever questions they have had along the way," says Lisa.

Kandy and Chris explained everything to their three-year-old girl from the very start and involved her in the events.

"She didn't know too much different," says Chris. "She didn't know you're supposed to have babies only for your family."

"I've been baby-sitting for other people's children quite a bit, so it was not a new thing for her that I took care of other people's children," says Kandy. "When I was going to have the transfer, I told her, 'Well, do you think the baby is going to stay this time?' After the baby stuck, she was very involved in it. She gave the baby hugs and kisses through my tummy, and she would tell the baby goodnight.

"When I was ready to go to the hospital, she was really excited. She said, 'We're going to the office to get the baby out.' She knew what was going on, and when the baby left there was no trouble."

Joy Parson, a divorced surrogate living in Maryland, delivered a surrogate baby in February 1986, when the oldest of her three children, Jack, was seven.

"He wasn't quite sure about me having this baby and not bringing it home. I think it gave him a little bit of a fear that he was going to go, too. But he has since realized that he is not going anywhere. He is here to stay with Mommy for good. I think he in time got more secure with it. Also he does see a counselor—he started long before."

Joy, who is about to be remarried to a man the children call Daddy, is a surrogate for the second time.

"When I had the last one, I said to the children that I was probably going to do it again, and Jack said, 'Well, I want my own baby.' When she explained she was not ready to have a baby of her own, Jack acquiesced.

Elizabeth Kane, the wife of an executive, gave birth to a surrogate baby six years ago. She was then an ardent supporter of the practice but has since changed her mind, partly because of her daughter's reaction. Her daughter is now seventeen, but, Kane told a *New York Times* reporter, "She is still having problems with what I did, and as a result she is still angry with me. Nobody told me that a child could bond with a baby while you're still pregnant. I didn't realize then that all the times she listened to his heartbeat and felt his legs kick that she was becoming attached to him."[5]

A 1985 Noel Keane surrogate, Peggy Pressler of Canton, Ohio, arranged ahead of time with the couple, Sally and Everett, for permission to keep in contact with the child, Adam. To her own daughter, Taylor, it was a bit confusing. She came home from school one day and asked, "Is Adam my brother?" Mrs. Pressler answered, "Yes, he's sort of your brother. He's Mommy's baby, but he's Sally's son, and he lives with Sally and Everett."

Mrs. Pressler, who is herself adopted, thought "it would be important for [Adam] to understand what happened, and to know who I was. I was pretty much in the dark when I grew up, and it only made everything more confusing to me."[6]

There are no studies on how a surrogate's own children react when a baby is given away.

"The only research that I'm aware of is sitting right here on my desk and that's very, very little," says Hilary Hanafin, who did a follow-up on her surrogates. Her report shows that the children have adjusted well and talk about it very little. But there are different responses at different ages.

"We are talking about children from age two to thirteen, so you are going to see a wide variety of responses. The older child has many more concerns about peers, about teachers, about how mom looks to friends and society. For the younger children it is much less important. Three- and four-year-olds tend to deal with it in a very resilient style. They are mostly happy that mom is not bringing the baby home and threatening their territory."

Only when the surrogate's children want a brother or sister do problems sometimes arise, according to Hanafin.

Reactions From Extended Family and Strangers

Surrogates do not just have to think of their own children, they have to be prepared for the reactions of family and friends and even total strangers.

Surrogate mother Elizabeth Kane was accused by her parents of giving away their grandchild, and schoolmates taunted her children. Another young surrogate in Maryland was forced to move out of her parents' home to an apartment elsewhere because of community antagonism.

Lisa Waters was especially concerned with the reaction of her father, "a strict person who has his own ideas about everything," but he "came through with flying colors." With her husband, Don's, parents, it was an entirely different story.

"They were very very angry about it, and that caused a few problems," says Lisa with diplomatic understatement. "I never found out what they didn't like about it, because they refused to allow me to speak about it. They just jumped all over me and decided that I was a terrible person."

Although her children were her in-laws' only grandchildren, they cut off the whole family for a while and put a great deal of pressure on Don.

"It was like: 'Come to your senses and leave this horrible woman, or you're not going to see us again,' " says Lisa.

Don's parents are still angry at Lisa months after the baby's birth. They will not speak to her, so when the family goes to Duluth, where both sets of grandparents live, Don and the children stay with his parents, and Lisa stays with her folks. She has learned to live with the situation.

"They are just people who feel they know what's right for everybody, and everybody should do what they say or they are not worth dealing with. I guess I have to feel sorry for them," she says with resignation.

On the other hand, Lisa got support from total strangers.

"When people found out about it, they were coming up to me and kissing me and saying that this was the best thing in the world. What was pretty amazing was the response from people who didn't even know me. My little hometown weekly paper had an article about me, and the next day I got flowers from somebody I didn't even know and a note saying, 'I think what you're doing is wonderful and I hope everything goes well for you.' I expected a lot more negative reaction, but didn't get it."

Kandy, too, had to answer a few questions. Her grandmother was upset.

"She is a very devout, religious person who thought this was adultery," says Kandy. "I asked her if it was adultery with him or with her or both. She couldn't see it, and it really bothered her."

One of Kandy's male acquaintances was vehemently against it.

"He just went on and on about how immoral, how wrong this was," says Kandy. "I had a hard time listening to him, because he was a father who wasn't married to the woman who had his child, and he was not supporting the child, just leeching off the mother. Just a very immoral, unkind person."

Kandy got a lot of support from her church.

"I go to a Lutheran church that is sixty percent widows over sixty, very conservative, and when I told them, they were all so loving, so nice: 'Oh, isn't it wonderful? What a beautiful thing to happen.' They were praying for the baby all the way, and the Sunday I was in the hospital having the baby, the pastor included us in the prayers."

Pregnancy and Birth

Many surrogates have been through pregnancy before and know what discomforts pregnancy entails, but the psychological circumstances are quite different when carrying a surrogate baby. How do you feel when a baby that is not yours starts to make its presence felt in your womb?

Kandy was thrilled. "I would say, 'Oh, oh, it's moving,' and I got so excited. I just never got tired of it." But Chris's reaction was less enthusiastic. "With our own daughter, he was always singing to her through my stomach and talking to her a lot. With this baby he didn't. He wasn't as interested.''

It requires determination not to get attached to the little human being in the womb.

"It's all mental," says Kandy, who chose to be an *in vitro* surrogate because, she says, "I didn't want to put myself through the experience of giving up a child that was genetically mine." But still, "I went through everything a genetic mother would . . . It is such a psychological thing of how you prepare yourself. I thought about it a lot, and I talked about it.''

Lisa Waters decided from the start not to think of the baby as hers "in any way, shape, or form.''

"I knew from the very first that it wasn't my baby, and I still feel that very strongly. I carried her; I know she was genetically half mine, but she is no way my baby. I didn't plan her. She would never have been born if her parents hadn't planned her, so I didn't have a problem.''

Statistics show that surrogates enjoy being pregnant, and that is indeed often the reason for their having babies for others. But no two pregnancies are alike, and none is risk-free.

"Pregnancy has its risks," Dr. Levitt points out. "You inform the patient, they understand the risks, and if they are willing to undergo the risks of pregnancy, it's their choice. I don't go into all the risks of pregnancy. There are too many." As a matter of fact, "pregnancy can kill you through a number of ways," adds Levitt, "but I don't say that.''

It almost killed Maria, a Michigan surrogate. Maria, with two children of her own, is a ballet instructor and a "health nut" who had no reason to anticipate problems.

"She was sitting at home one evening, watching TV," recounts Carmen Dubois, the mother of the child Maria gave birth to, "and suddenly her placenta tears away. Maria's husband rushed her to the nearest hospital. She was dying from the loss of blood.'' Clinically she was dead—twice, but she was revived and survived. After three weeks in the hospital both she and her healthy baby were discharged.

Kandy's difficulties seem insignificant by comparison. Kandy explains, "With this [surrogate] baby I was swelling a lot. I gained fifty-five pounds. I was just round. I had carpal tunnel syndrome, and that means that I was swelling so badly that I was pinching a nerve in my wrist. It was my right hand naturally, so there I was with my left hand, bathing my daughter, cooking, and doing dishes. Just everything was difficult.''

Larry got extremely worried. "They scared me," he says. "The agency called and said, 'It sounds as if she is getting too bloated and that she could be in real serious trouble.' "

The doctor ordered Kandy to stay in bed for at least five hours a day during the very last part of the pregnancy.

Childbirth is painful, even in the easiest of deliveries, but Katie Abrams' delivery was a real horror story.

After a 1986 Thanksgiving dinner at her mother's house, Katie went into labor. Her water broke, and slight contractions started. She got to the hospital around 7:00 o'clock the next morning but was still only in mild labor. At 11:00 o'clock the doctors decided to give her Pitocin intravenously to induce labor. By 2:00 in the afternoon, her cervix was 90 percent dilated, and Katie was asked to start pushing the baby out.

"They had me push and push and push for the next two hours. They had me stand in bed to push, they had me squat, they had me in every position they could think of. I was really uncomfortable," she says.

By 6:00 o'clock the baby had moved up instead of down, and the doctor was called away on an emergency. When he got back half an hour later, the pushing resumed, but still no baby.

"The doctor looked at me real funny. I said, 'What's wrong?' He said, 'Nothing. It's fine. Don't worry about it.' "

Katie was exhausted and, because of the way she "felt inside," she knew that a cesarean section was in the offing. She was put to sleep and the doctors delivered a normal boy. Katie, however, was so swollen inside from all the fruitless pushing that the doctor "couldn't even get a catheter up there." The hospital kept her packed in ice for three days—"I was completely numb." People told her "she was made of steel," but the compliments did not cheer her up, she was upset.

Giving Up Baby

The delivery may be hard, but, one would imagine, the hardest part, saying goodbye to the newborn, is still to come. A surprising number of surrogates report no difficulties giving up the baby. Like Dee, who had a baby for Carol and Peter Wright, and Janet Reid, Lisa Waters suffered no emotional torment relinquishing the girl she gave birth to in February 1987.

"The day after she was born, a nurse brought her to my room and I spent about a half hour with her. From the first moment I saw her I felt, 'Here is a baby of some dear friends. She is beautiful, strong and healthy and I'm so happy for them.' Honestly, I didn't feel she was mine at all.''

Katie, too, did not find it hard to give up the baby, because "my energies towards the baby were always that this is not my child." But she was disappointed, to say the least, about her treatment after the delivery.

"In the hospital I couldn't get any information about the baby from [the agency people] as to the weight and time of birth. Finally I asked the nurses, and they gave it to me. That's information I need."

Katie has not heard from the parents since the birth—not even a thank-you note—which bothers her, because she just wants to know that the baby is all right—"Once I know, I don't have any problems with it."

She does not miss the baby, but she has kept a journal for the boy "just in case he ever looks for me. I'm not dreaming that he will. They are not baby-sitting. He is their child. I did it a lot for myself and . . . I just wanted to be assured that if he ever finds out that he is a surrogate child there will be no confusion as to why I did what I did." One of her entries says to the child, "Please don't ever be ashamed of your beginnings. Realize that your parents were willing to sacrifice anything. They loved you and wanted you so much that they would have given up their lives for you. And don't feel bad for what I did. I could see how much they wanted a child."

Kandy's couple was very concerned about her emotional well-being after the delivery and would not leave until they knew she was all right. They even suggested that she come home with them, but she was fine.

Kandy's husband, though, suffered a letdown right after the birth. Says Chris, "It was like, hey, Kandy is working so hard to have that baby, and it was like *we* were having a baby. I was in there beside her, coaching her through the whole thing. So after it was all over—wow, all that work! A baby! And yet we don't have a baby. I felt like walking down the hallway, jumping up and clicking my heels, but then thinking, 'But we don't have it.' There was kind of a void there for maybe an hour. I was a little confused, but then it all came together again."

When the couple left with the baby, Kandy had "a sense of love," but when they were gone, "all of a sudden I got this feeling that I was missing her," Kandy says, "and I cried and cried. That feeling of sadness lasted for three days, and that was it."

"Kandy is the Rock of Gibraltar," says Chris. "She is incredible."

Kandy still has a lot of contact with the couple, and the wife is "like a sister" to Kandy. "We are very close, and I would love to do it for them again."

Donna Regan, who has been a surrogate twice, is a pro. She had no trouble giving up the first baby.

"You go into the surrogate parenting program knowing that that's what the outcome is going to be. To expect anything different would have been naïve. I knew it wasn't going to be easy, but it was easier than I had even anticipated."

During the first pregnancy she had stuck strictly to her own mental rules about not breast-feeding and set limits to the amount of contact with the future parents. The second time she became pregnant with twins.

"I knew I could allow myself to go a lot further emotionally than I had the first time. I let myself get a lot closer, not only to the couple but to the babies before and after they were born. So it was a little more difficult, but it was somewhat more rewarding in the end. It really turned out to be something much more fulfilling than the first time even." Apparently, a lot of it, if not all, is in the mind.

These particular surrogates may be a "special breed of women," as one adoptive mother of a surrogate baby expressed it, but Hilary Hanafin's studies of surrogates seem to indicate that they are the norm rather than the exception.

"I have never had a surrogate change her mind, and I have never had a surrogate tell me that she regretted the decision to become a surrogate." In fifty-five surrogate births, Hanafin "can only think of two cases where there was any kind of grieving over the child. There can be grieving, but grieving over the child is almost never seen. Sometimes surrogates grieve over the loss of the role of being a surrogate, which is a very special and psychologically satisfying role for them. Sometimes it is grieving over the fact that they can't decide what to do with their lives after being a surrogate. There are lots of feelings, but rarely do they revolve around a simple loss regarding the child."

Are surrogates who don't grieve over the child cold and calculating women?

Lori Andrews, a lawyer with the American Bar Foundation, who has met and talked to a large number of surrogates, has found surrogates "to be very loving and very special. A woman has to be altruistic and sensitive to the needs of the infertile in order to be a surrogate . . . The pregnant surrogate lovingly talks to and sings to the baby inside her, just as any pregnant woman does. She bonds to the baby, but she does so in a different way.''[7]

Says Hanafin, "Society tells them there must be something wrong with them, when the exact opposite is true. They are usually incredibly sensitive and empathetic moral women for whom motherhood is everything, but people are real suspicious of them because they can give up a baby."

Psychologist Dennis Harrison thinks that a surrogate "probably has the ability to emotionally cut off across the board. I've seen one surrogate in particular with her three-year-old. She could be so detached about the child she was carrying, and with her own child she was warm and open and talked to everybody about it."

As Hanafin suggests, handing over the child to the parents it was destined for represents more than leaving the baby. While a surrogate is pregnant, she is a "precious person" who basks in both positive and negative attention, is often featured in newspaper articles, and appears on television. Kandy went on television a couple of times, and as her husband, Chris, says, "Anybody I talked with, it was, 'Wow, she is really being somebody, being a neat person doing that.' "

The surrogate is in the thoughts and wishes of the future parents to whom she is temporarily the most important person in the world, which they often let her know through letters and gifts, and she feels grand about her power to make several people deliriously happy. As Lisa Waters realized when she got a beautiful letter from the parents "that made everybody cry, I wasn't just helping create a baby, or even a mom and a dad; I was creating grandparents, aunts and uncles, a whole network of people who wouldn't have known these types of relationships if I hadn't entered the program."

When the baby goes, everything else often disappears with it. Correspondence from the parents may cease completely or dwindle to a few cards a year. Says Barbara Delsanto, "It's kind of like they forget what you've done." The surrogate faces normal postpartum depression without a baby to keep her busy and for admiring relatives to coo over, and then it's back to everyday life. When she says goodbye to the baby, she says hello to a life of ordinariness, while the baby is still the focal point of all her feelings.

Dennis Harrison suggests to surrogates that they have a private little ceremony to say goodbye to the baby. "They shouldn't just hurry themselves through the goodbyes. It is a very personal thing how they do it. It really gets down to this: 'I'm doing it for this couple, and have a good life. Goodbye.' And they cry a little bit. Usually the doctor will leave the baby with them for a while, and we talk about it ahead of time. They know they have the right up until the paper is signed to get out of the room, walk over to the maternity ward, and pick up the baby.''

The baby M case may have given the impression that surrogates are inclined to do that, but only four or five out of over 500 have done so. But there are surrogates who keep longing for the baby for extended periods of time.

For surrogate Elizabeth, who gave birth to a son for a Colorado couple in 1983 at the age of thirty-one, the decision to give up the child looked different before and after the moment of separation. She had been determined to try surrogate motherhood and was very happy for the adoptive mother when she became pregnant with the husband's sperm. After the delivery of the baby, at which the couple was present, she felt it was more their baby than hers, but during the adoption proceedings the floodgates opened, and she started to cry. At the airport she gave the baby one last hug.

"The saddest goodbye," she said. "Turning away from the baby was the hardest thing I've ever done in my life. I didn't look back. I knew if I did I might not be able to handle it. It was the saddest goodbye I've ever known, even though I had told myself again and again during the pregnancy that it was not really my baby. The tears refused to stop. I cried for three days after I got home. Finally, on Easter Sunday, Susan [the adoptive mother] called me from Denver. She said, 'I lie here with the baby on my chest, watching him sleep, and, Elizabeth, I feel he is now my own.' Only then was I able to stop crying.''[8]

Barbara Delsanto felt very tempted to do what Mary Beth Whitehead did. She gave birth to a surrogate girl in August 1986. Two weeks before the birth, she started "feeling bad." Her delivery was easy—three hours. She held the baby as soon as it was born, and she did not let the nurses separate them. "I'm not leaving," she said, "I'm going to stay right here with the baby." She cared for the baby in the hospital for two days, but then the moment of truth arrived.

"I cried. I cried really hard. I told her I loved her and always would, and that she would always be in my heart, but that she belonged to them, not me.''

Bending all agency rules, Barbara insisted on seeing the parents, and when she saw them with the baby through the window in the nursery, "I started crying more; but just looking at them, I could tell that they really wanted her, that she was a long awaited gift."

The first week after the departure of the baby was "truly hell."

"It was the postpartum blues," Barbara thinks. "I said, 'Oh God, what have I done. Oh God, I love her so much.' "

Her husband and mother-in-law kept reminding her of "what I was doing and why I was doing it." She went home to her parents and cried with her mother. "I guess within a month or two I felt a lot better."

Although Barbara is "not that type of person," she was close to changing her mind about giving up the baby.

"If I could have had a chance to get my baby back, I probably would have done the same thing as Mary Beth Whitehead, but my husband let me cry and I had some tranquilizers that I took once or twice a day when I thought I was going to get really upset."

A year later, Barbara still misses her baby, but she is not ruling out being a surrogate again if the parents want a sibling for their daughter.

The Money Issue

Once the surrogate has signed the papers relinquishing the baby, she receives her fee for services rendered—usually around $10,000.

"People ask me why surrogates get ten thousand dollars," says Hanafin. "She spends nine months being pregnant, and in our program a surrogate spends over two hundred hours in medical appointments: workups, inseminations, prenatal examinations, labor and delivery, legal and psychological appointments. They spend three hours a month with a psychologist—it is mandatory—and all the surrogates have to attend the surrogate support group meetings from the time they apply until two months postpartum. It is not a quick nine months."

To many surrogates the compensation is an important incentive but hardly ever, they say, the only one.

When Barbara Delsanto signed up with Infertility Associates International in Maryland, she was not aware that she would be paid.

"I never heard of anybody getting paid to do it. I said, 'You mean I'm getting paid for this?' In fact I was shocked. I thought they were going to help with the medical expenses. I thought that's what the money was for."

Barbara and her husband were buying a house, so she accepted the money—"It came in handy."

Ian Sutton, a nurse in California who has given birth to two surrogate babies at the age of thirty-three and thirty-four, claims that the money was not a factor in her decision.

"The money really wasn't all that much, and I would have done it anyway simply for the cost. What I was involved in was the excitement of what I was doing. I remembered how excited I had made one family with our own children and so I wanted to do the same for somebody who couldn't have children."[9]

She "blew" the money on a trip to Hawaii.

Lisa Waters has this to say about the fee: "It meant a lot in that it represented that I was performing a service for someone who couldn't perform it. In other words, I felt I was doing a job. But beyond that the money wasn't at all a motivation. It was like, gee, it's sort of nice that I'm getting this too, and I certainly didn't turn it down. But it wasn't the prime motivating factor. I would have done it without being paid."

She does not consider $10,000 a lot of money for the service she performed.

"If you figure it out, the number of hours one is pregnant during a full-term pregnancy, it is a little under a dollar an hour—not much of a payment for a job."

Lisa paid off some loans and banked a good chunk of the money, "knowing that the government will take it away from us at the end of the year."

Kandy Harris was inspired to become a surrogate after giving birth to her own child.

"I thought the birth of my daughter was so exciting, so miraculous, it was so wonderful. I thought if I could do that for somebody else I would. The money was critical in that that was why I was willing to do it for somebody I didn't have an emotional attachment to. I had an aunt and an uncle that I did offer to do this for previously. I said if he quit smoking I would have their baby for them, but they suddenly got pregnant—with twins! But doing it for somebody you don't know, I think it is reasonable to be paid." But "if I were doing it for the money—not that I would—it is not enough money to do it."

Even couples who have to pay do not feel that surrogates are getting very much.

"Not at all," says Lorna Gallo, the mother of surrogate baby Annie. "I know I could never do it."

Anita Cody, the mother of surrogate baby Brian, says, "I don't think there is any woman alive who would spend a year and a half for another couple for nothing," so the payment of $10,000 "doesn't seem a lot to me." On second thought, Anita remarks, "It's about right, because she was able to continue her job, so it didn't cramp her lifestyle." But Anita feels "it's outrageous" that the surrogate agency is paid the same amount—and sometimes more—than the mother.

Paying surrogates to bear children for others has many people upset. To many it seems immoral.

Says Hanafin, "If you took the money away from surrogacy, people would still not like it, but the money has really tainted it."

Because surrogates accept money, cynics tend to doubt surrogates' humanitarian impulses. Take, for instance, Michael Kinsey, the editor of the *New Republic*. He thinks that people "who deny the commercial nature of the transaction (who say surrogate mothers are doing it out of love, and not for money) are being coy." But he and others are then at a loss to explain why surrogates would put themselves through so much for so little, if, as he says, "no one is forcing women to do this."[10]

Critics of surrogacy point out that the number of surrogate mothers willing to work for Noel Keane's operation dropped off to virtually nothing when it appeared that Michigan laws made it illegal to pay a mother who was giving up a surrogate or any other child for adoption. Noel Keane tried to have the law overturned, and during the case the attorney for the state argued that "the primary purpose of this money is to encourage women to volunteer to be surrogate mothers."

Well, of course it is. Attorneys do not become attorneys for purely altruistic reasons either. And how come doctors whose main concern supposedly is to help people often make disgraceful amounts of money?

The Exploitation Issue

Strangely enough, at the very same time that the general public is outraged that surrogates mix babies with business, it also worries about surrogates being poor exploited women. From an altruistic standpoint surrogates seem calculating. From a business standpoint they seem exploited.

When surrogacy first came to the attention of the general public in the 1970s, ethicist Leon Kass predicted in an article in the

Journal of the American Medical Association that only prostitutes would agree to become surrogates. Other pundits were sure that only very poor women would be willing to put their bodies on the line, that surrogacy would lead to the exploitation of poor women by wealthy couples. That has not turned out to be the case. Prostitutes would be unlikely to take a cut in income, and besides, they would be screened out by the agencies that match couples with surrogates.

Although there have been no examples of millionaires acting as surrogate mothers for a couple on welfare, Noel Keane had a Jewish lawyer give birth to a child for a rabbi, and one Chicago career woman signed up with an agency as a surrogate. She wanted the $10,000 so she could have a nanny for her own child, but she skipped out on the scheduled insemination when her father threatened to disown her. Surrogates are not heiresses, but they are not necessarily poor women.

Women on welfare need not apply as surrogates to Surrogate Motherhood, Inc., in Laurel, Maryland. They will not even be considered.

Says Matthew Myers, attorney for the agency, "We have a balancing act in picking surrogates. It is essential from our point of view that people who become surrogates do so freely and voluntarily. If the money we are going to pay them is the difference between their survival and nonsurvival, the ability to feed their families or not, I think there are some potentially strong questions as to how free the choice really is. They are in a position where they are desperate for money, and in that circumstance there is at least an argument that they haven't entered into it as freely as possible. There is also an argument that we are using and abusing their poverty to take advantage of their bodies. We don't want surrogacy to be an upper class use of lower class women to produce their offspring."

Hilary Hanafin agrees. "It seems bad politics to accept women who are in dire need of financial assistance, and for women on welfare, the case could be made that they are doing it purely for the money. Secondly, if a woman is on welfare, she is bound and obligated to tell the government about any other funds she is receiving, so for most of them it doesn't make sense."

Of course, there are always less ethical operators. Dr. Howard Adelman, a psychologist for Surrogate Mothering Ltd. in Philadelphia, which as of this writing is on its way out of business, told *Ob/Gyn News*, "I believe candidates with an element of financial need are the safest. If a woman is on unemployment and has children to care for, she is not likely to change her mind and want to keep the baby she is being paid to have for somebody else."[11]

Over the last decade, thousands of women have applied to become surrogates, enough for professional psychologists to begin to look for trends in the surrogate population.

"Means and Standard Deviations of Demographic Characteristics of Surrogate Volunteers" is the heading of a table of statistics on surrogate candidates. It was part of a handout that Dr. Joan Einwohner distributed when she presented a paper entitled "Surrogate Motherhood: Motivations and Dynamics" at the New York State Psychological Association in April 1987.

Dr. Einwohner, who screens candidates for the Infertility Institute of New York City, found the mean age of those she interviewed was 26.3, their mean intelligence was 99.8, and the mean number of children they already had was 1.5. They were housewives, bookkeepers, counselors, managers, secretaries, teachers, switchboard operators, technicians, farmers, etc.—a variety of backgrounds that do not lend themselves to easy generalizations. On the sheet of motivational statistics, "money" and "enjoying being pregnant" were at the top of the list. Other categories included were "desire to experience pregnancy" and "sympathy for childlessness," as well as "regret for abortion." These people, while perhaps not the most sophisticated members of society, can hardly be characterized as lost souls.

Nevertheless, many feminists—Barbara Katz Rothman, for instance—fear exploitation of poor women. Rothman believes that a $10,000 payment for nine months' work, twenty-four hours a day, entailing substantial physical and emotional transformation [is] a figure that would only tempt women for whom work has always been a dead-end, as it is for so many working-class women."[12]

This is an attitude that insults surrogates.

Surrogate Donna Regan, who has an I.Q. that more than qualifies her for Mensa, is angry: "I'm not poor, and I'm certainly not stupid. I'm not in any manner ignorant or uneducated, so there is really no basis for argument there. None of the surrogates I have ever met have been stupid or uneducated. If you get right down to it, if you don't have a lot of money, or if you are not highly educated, it shouldn't mean that you're less capable of making a choice."

When a group of women talked to Donna Regan about surrogates being low class, she was "terribly offended."—"My family would certainly not be called low class."

Surrogate Dee, whose husband, Dale, owns his own refrigeration business, does not like that kind of talk either, but she has heard it before.

"Yes, 'poor women having babies for rich ones.' I hate it when I hear that. I'm not rich by any means, but I'm certainly not on skid row either, and the money I made was not a major factor. A lot of couples who come into this program have obviously saved every dime they can get their hands on, so I hate that scenario of poor women having babies for rich women."

There may be ample reason to distrust testimony from directors of surrogacy agencies, but since they have dealt with a large number of surrogates, they may be worth listening to.

Beth Bacon, one such administrator, asserts that surrogates "don't like to be seen as victims, as these pathetic creatures who have no brains of their own and no options. They are offended when people imply that they are helpless creatures being exploited."

To psychologist Hilary Hanafin, a dues-paying member of NOW, "it is a disappointment to see these feminist organizations come to their conclusions without ever talking to surrogate mothers. Women casting other women in a role without ever speaking to them, I think, is rather embarrassing. I don't want their opinions unless they have done their homework."

Does Kenda Harris, who had to abstain from normal sex for ten months, who went through three painful embryo transfers, who gained fifty-five pounds and suffered from carpal tunnel syndrome, who only got $8,500 in compensation, feel exploited?

"Never! Never, never, never," she says. "I think it's a lot of baloney. I did something out of my own free will that I felt good about. It has increased my self-esteem—I felt like Mother Earth. It is part of giving life, it was wonderful. In no way do I feel exploited."

Does Janet Reid feel exploited?

"No, I don't feel exploited at all. The feminists are the ones denigrating women, saying that they don't know what they are doing, saying that we are mindless. I wanted to do what I did," she insists.

Rather than feeling exploited by infertile women, many surrogates feel an emotional bond with them.

Says Barbara Delsanto, "When I heard that some women were against surrogacy, I was quite shocked, because here we are, women helping other women. If you want to be fighting, there are a lot of other things to be fighting against, like pornography—to me, *that's* exploiting a woman's body."

Lisa Waters' felt a connection with the infertile wife.

"I know from myself what it is to be a mother, so I was relating to her. Plus she did all the letter writing."

In a gesture that hardly becomes an exploited woman, Lisa sent half a dozen roses to the wife on Mother's Day.

"I wanted to do something special for her, because I wanted her to feel it was *her* Mother's Day."

Says Dee, "The main thing is between the women, for each woman to accept the other. I can give her what she wants, and she can have from me what I can give her. I think it takes a very admirable woman to accept that she has to go through another woman." But Dee also feels a connection with the husband. "I'll look at a picture of him and the baby, and I think there is a jointness between the three of us."

By their own admission, the money surrogates receive for their services is not a lot. But, they also have altruistic motives for doing it, such as helping other women. Why won't we believe them?

"The belief that the good fortune of others is also finally one's own does not come easily or invariably to the human breast," says George Gilder, the supply-side guru and author of *Wealth and Poverty*.[13] The general public has a hard time grasping it, but it seems that both surrogates and the couples they have babies for operate precisely on that principle. They, like the rest of us, live in a capitalistic society, and they would probably believe Gilder when he claims that the essence of capitalism is not greed but giving.

Surrogate mothers are not true supply-siders, since they do not let supply create its own demands; they fill a need already there. Infertile people want babies, and surrogate mothers produce them. They understand the needs of others and fill them in what many people think is a surprising way. But, as we all know, "[one] does not make gifts without some sense, possibly unconscious, that one will be rewarded, whether in this world or the next. Even the biblical injunction affirms that the giver will be given unto," says Gilder.[14]

The gift of the couple, their investment, is the money; the surrogate's gift is a baby.

"Capitalist production entails faith—in one's neighbors, in one's society, and in the compensatory logic of the cosmos," but it does not rule out "the awesome uncertainties and commensurate acts of faith that are indispensable to an expanding and innovative system.[15] . . . These gifts or investments are experimental in that the returns to the giver are unknown; and whether gains or losses, they are absorbed by him,'' says Gilder.[16]

The couple may lose their investment—and some have. They may end up with a stillborn or defective child. Surrogates may go through a lot of agony and not get paid if they miscarry, and they may get no appreciation from the couple if everything else goes well, so that at the end they may well feel that the reward was not commensurate with their effort or suffering. As with all transactions, there are definitely uncertainties on both sides.

Those who think that surrogates are being exploited have to understand that surrogates do not get their reward in only one currency. They have to buy groceries, so they like part of their reward in dollars, but since they, unlike many businessmen, recognize values beyond money, they can take their reward in terms of personal satisfaction that comes from having done something a bit heroic and from knowing they have fulfilled someone's dream.

It is not surprising that the United States is the only country in the world where paid surrogacy has become such a phenomenon— after all, both parents and surrogates are products of the society they live in. What is amazing is that surrogate mothers are not pushing for more money. Says Gloria Steinem, ''. . .if men could give birth, they'd be charging a million dollars—and they'd have a cartel.''[17]

Obviously surrogates are not ''baby barons''; perhaps they are capitalists with a female face and female values.

The Myth of the Passive Barren Wife

It does not come as a surprise that feminists think that men, whose selfish genes want to be perpetuated, are the prime exploiters, not just of the surrogates but of their wives. Gloria Steinem once remarked, ''What seems to come first in the cases I've read about is an obsession with sperm and paternity. . . . ''[18]

Not so, according to Beth Bacon. ''Sometimes you'll hear, 'Well, this guy is on an ego trip and he's got to have his own sperm and he's got to have his own baby, and his wife is sitting over there, thrown aside like a piece of barren luggage.' But that is not the case. Usually it is the wife who calls us, the wife who tells the husband, 'Let's enroll. I want a baby. I really want your child.

I really want to do this.' It is not the husband dragging along this poor woman who is feeling inadequate.''

This is how the parents of surrogate babies answer the question who wanted the baby?

Marilyn Smith: ''I probably have to say me.''

Lorna Gallo: ''I divorced my first husband. He didn't really care that I couldn't get pregnant.'' What about her second husband? ''He didn't desperately want children.''

Anita Cody: ''I think it was both. It wasn't one or the other.''

Carol Wright: ''It was my initial idea. I dragged my husband into it initially, but it didn't take long for him to jump on the bandwagon. But at first it was my idea.''

Peter Wright: ''My wife was always the thorough researcher in our family, and when she came through with this, I knew it was the answer.''

The first couple in the United States to have a surrogate baby were George and Debbie.

Says George, ''I told Debbie that I married her because I loved her, not because I wanted children. I was perfectly content to live our lives just the way we were.''

Debbie observes, ''All I ever wanted from life was to get married and have children. That was my dream and I never stopped believing in it. I grew up fighting for what I believe in.''[12]

Only Carmen Dubois, who already had a grown daughter from a previous marriage, does not fit the pattern—''Mainly I was pleasing my husband at the time, but it has changed.''

Let's hear from the experts. Who instigates surrogate procedures?

Dr. Dennis Harrison, a forensic psychologist and consultant to Surrogate Motherhood, Inc., of Laurel, Maryland, says, ''I would probably say the wife. The wife sees something on TV or reads something about it, and they ease into it.''

Dr. Joan Einwohner, a psychologist and consultant to the Infertility Institute in New York City, replies, ''It is usually the infertile wife who drags her husband to the clinic. She has tried and tried to have children the usual way. She wants to have a child, to get on with it. Most of the surrogates have the fantasy of handing the baby to the woman who needs a child. The men are surprisingly irrelevant in this.''

Surrogacy and Feminism

Infertility may be on the rise, but it is not a new phenomenon. Childless couples desperate for a baby have always availed themselves of every possible opportunity to get a child of their own. Medically, surrogacy, as practiced today, has been possible ever since the techniques of artificial insemination were developed a century ago. So why was it not considered a viable option for infertile couples until recently? The medical capability has been available for a long time, but the social climate did not allow it. What has changed?

In some respects, apparently not much. Infertile women and surrogates seem to be two sides of the "eternally feminine," to use a romantic expression. Many women feel that one, if not the most important, role in their lives is to be a mother, and surrogates express—granted, in a new way—another old female tradition: self-sacrifice, putting other people's interests ahead of their own in an attempt to relieve unhappiness in the world.

Joan Field, a surrogate with two children of her own, expresses the female selflessness. "I did something in the past that made me really aware of this need that I have to feel that way. I donated milk to the Mothers' Milk Bank. I was supplying milk to several premature babies in the hospital. I realized that I like this feeling of doing something personal for people. Being a surrogate is something I can do. I add to the real happiness in the world, true happiness."

And surrogate Lisa Waters, once a member of NOW, was inspired by a similar impulse. "I feel God has given me so much, what can I give back? I knew I would never do anything wonderful like ending our nuclear arms race, but I knew this was one of the best things I could do." And now, she says, "I've made my statement, given my gift."

"'We were brought up in my family to think that if you needed something from me and there wasn't any reason in the world that I shouldn't give it to you, then I should go ahead and help you," says Donna Regan. "I grew up on an author that put out a book called *Time Enough for Love*. I always felt that if I didn't have that much to give to somebody else, I wasn't worth a hell of a lot as a person. Think what a tiny bit of the whole picture you're looking at it is to take time out of my life to give somebody else a child. It doesn't even compare."

Women have traditionally been brought up to believe that their greatest contributions to the world are as nurturers, helpers, even martyrs. To some people, especially feminists, such self-sacrificing impulses are suspect. It is a sign of a low self-image, they argue. Sick.

It is interesting that an apparently disproportional number of surrogates have been brought up in the Catholic church, which more than any other Christian group encourages self-sacrifice. Among the surrogates appearing in this book, Janet Reid, Barbara Delsanto, Joan Field, and Mary Beth Whitehead were brought up as Catholics. Philip Parker, a psychologist at Wayne State University, found that in a group of 120 surrogate applicants, 69 were Protestant, 50 were Catholic, and 1 was Jewish. In Hilary Hanafin's group of surrogates, one-third was Catholic, still a larger percentage than Catholics in the general population, which is around 25 percent. It is ironic that the Catholic church, which condemns surrogacy, fosters the impulses that inspire women to become surrogate mothers.

It is true that many surrogates mention that helping others by giving them a baby has enhanced their self-respect, but that is not the same as saying that they did not have any before they got into surrogacy. Probably all human beings continually seek to enhance their self-respect through their relationships, work, and beliefs. Just because surrogates enhance their self-image in a uniquely feminine way does not in and of itself make it a new form of mental derangement. Undoubtedly, there are surrogates with critically low self-esteem, who are confused about the proper role of women, but all of the surrogates who speak in this book appear to be unusually strong, independent women able to take a lot of abuse without crumbling. If they are confused about their actions, they hide it extremely well. Not one has asked for sympathy or approval, and all want to be considered capable, rational beings, not as feckless creatures who need protection from feminists and other well-meaning people.

Says Donna Regan, "For years the feminist movement, from its inception really, has supported the idea that as a woman you have the right to make your own decisions, that you are not any less capable because you're female. I'm an extraordinarily intelligent person. I'm very much aware of what I'm doing, and I resent the implication that I need someone else to tell me what I should be doing."

There is little doubt that surrogates are carrying on the female tradition of selflessness in a new way, but still they are violating the most fundamental aspect of a traditional woman's role. They are breaking the supposedly unbreakable bond with the children they give birth to. Something must have changed to make them feel free to do that.

Maybe the feminists who are so worried about surrogacy helped pave the way.

Hanafin's surrogates "are women—twenty-six, twenty-eight—who are not part of the feminist movement, but they reap the benefits of that and therefore feel comfortable saying, 'I am who I am, I don't have to follow anybody's rules.' Society has created a climate where women feel free to be surrogate mothers, when they never could have done it in the thirties and forties."

Feminists have long argued that women should not be prisoners of their biological destiny, and an important step in the liberation of women was abortion on demand. It gave them increased control of their bodies. They could choose *not* to bear a child without asking for anybody's permission.

Surrogacy is the opposite side of the coin. Surrogate mothers can choose to bear a child, at least in theory, without their husband's blessing, and some do. They are essentially saying, "My body is my own and I can do with it what I please, whether I am married or single. Nobody owns my body except me." It seems strange to find feminists now accusing surrogates, who have not only risen above their destiny but turned it into a source of income, of turning back the clock in some ways.

Is surrogacy a trap that feminists have uncovered? Are surrogates playing into the hands of men?

Says Lori Andrews, "There is much divisiveness among feminists on the issue, but I think some are responding from a fairly well-grounded historical perspective that women have been denied custody of their children for all sorts of stereotypical reasons. Women's role in reproduction has been underrated in a sense. Until this century, men automatically got custody, children were the property of men, and surrogacy conjures up an image of men again being able to use women's bodies for their own ends. Of course, that creates this fear. I part company in the sense that I see surrogates as very strong, independent actors, and I don't see it as men taking control."

The Baby M case increased fears of women's losing control. Mary Beth Whitehead was abused in court and summarily deprived of the rights to her child with what seems inadequate legal justification. As a verdict in a straight custody case, it seems very unfair; in a contract dispute, quite reasonable.

While feminists may have some justified cause for concern,

those who are most opposed seem to base their objection to surrogacy soley on the Baby M case. Refusing to look beyond that tragic situation, they want to save everybody from the evils of surrogacy.

It is the feminists most strongly against surrogacy who are most often heard from, and apparently their view is gaining in academic circles.

Imagine the halls of Boston University filled with law students, predominantly women, who have come to listen to lawyers and surrogates explain what the practice is all about. There isn't an empty seat; the overflow crowd sits in the windowsills and on tables. Everybody wants to hear about surrogacy—the Baby M verdict has just been handed down. The press has turned out in force, too. The television cameras are rolling, and print journalists have their pens poised.

On the platform behind a table, sit the female moderator; George Annas, professor of law; and Herbert Brail from Noel Keane's office. Just below in the front row are two surrogate mothers, Laurie Johnson and Donna Regan.

The evening's first speaker, George Annas, is introduced. An expert on surrogacy from an intellectual point of view, he has written several scholarly papers on the practice, has testified before congressional committees, and his bespectacled, bearded face often appears in newpapers along with his sage comments.

As a professor of health law at Boston University, he has the home court advantage. His students are in the audience. He starts off in a sarcastic and somewhat condescending tone, as usual condemning surrogacy as abhorrent, particularly because the surrogates accept a fee. The crowd appears to enjoy the familiar expert denunciations.

The audience, mostly too young to worry about infertility, is well primed for the next speaker, attorney Herbert Brail, who occasionally handles surrogacy arrangements for Noel Keane. Not surprisingly, he speaks as an advocate of the practice, and expresses the opinion that perhaps the country should be more concerned about teenage pregnancy than surrogacy.

The crowd hisses.

The surrogates look at each other, astonished. Donna Regan wants to leave but is persuaded to stay by Laurie Johnson who is about to throw herself to the wolves.

Laurie is introduced as a Keane surrogate who is not married and has no children of her own. She speaks with a great deal of assurance about her reasons for getting into surrogacy and explains the process. The crowd is quiet. She is making an impression.

Donna is the last panelist. By the time her turn comes, the format has changed to questions and answers.

The perpetual question: "Why did you become a surrogate?"

"Because it is the most natural thing in the world for me to help somebody else," Donna answers.

The audience moans.

One woman concerned about genetic engineering wants to know what would have happened if the surrogate twins Donna recently gave birth to had had the "wrong" eye color? Also, given her extraordinarily high I.Q., was Donna out to populate the world with super-intelligent children?

Donna, dumbfounded, answers, "The parents didn't care, all they wanted was a child."

The woman was not really interested in an answer, and derogatory sounds from the background cut Donna's answer short.

Another woman asks how well Donna took care of herself during the pregnancy.

"I certainly took as good care of myself as I could. I felt a terrific responsibility carrying somebody else's child—"

Boos rise from the audience. The evening reminds Donna of a lynching party. All the questions are asked in a hostile way, and not a single person voices a word of support.

More questions, more hisses and boos.

The moderator concludes the evening's entertainment, and most of the audience begins to file out. It is now the press's turn to ask question of the panelists, but students and other interested participants stick around.

George Annas chats with Donna and confides that he doesn't really have a problem with surrogacy per se.

"What did I just hear you say?" asks a gentleman with long ears, and the television cameras zoom in on them.

"Well, no," George Annas says, "I don't want you to think I like what she did," and goes back into his professorial mode. Suddenly, after the official part of the evening is over, there are lots of women telling Donna that they can appreciate what she did. Some have relatives who can't have children, others are adoptees who feel strongly that surrogacy is a more open form of adoption, and so it goes. Publicly, of course, they dare not say this. In Professor Annas's department at Boston University, that is not kosher thinking.

Said Donna after the meeting, "I never felt such hostility and really intense dislike." She has run into a lot of people who don't approve of surrogacy, but never anything like the furies at Boston University. "The fact that I was willing to stand up there and talk about it does not give them the right to take pot shots at me. They don't have to agree with what I did—that's not important to me—but they have to respect that it was my choice to make."

Many feminists feel differently about it and are surprisingly emotional about the issue, and there are legitimate reasons to be concerned about abuses.

Says Hilary Hanafin, "There is certainly without a doubt the potential for exploitation; it is tremendous. I'm pleased that the feminist organizations have pointed out that possibility."

During the Baby M case, it was argued by feminists and many other well-meaning people that the contract a surrogate signs to give up the baby cannot and should not be enforced because there is no way the surrogate can know what she will feel once the baby is born, and therefore she cannot give "informed consent."

"You know, they didn't let women make contracts in Victorian days," says psychologist Joan Einwohner. "I think it is a throwback to Victorian days that a woman can't enter into a [surrogate] contract because she is considered so vulnerable to hormones and her emotions that she's like an irresponsible child and must be protected from herself."

Writer Mary Gordon has struggled with that issue.

"There is part of me that believes in the supremacy of keeping one's word, and that fears men will use against us the argument that a woman, under pressure of her emotional response to giving birth, cannot be expected to keep her word. For centuries men have claimed that women are not equal moral agents to men, that we are ruled by our bodies in ways men are not, and therefore we must be kept from that responsibility." Gordon, however, has come to the conclusion that with surrogacy, as with marriage vows, it is permissible to break one's word.[19]

"One of my prime concerns in this area as a feminist myself," says lawyer Lori Andrews, "is that the rationale we use to justify policy in this area be consistent and not come back to haunt us in other areas."

Every person who signs a contract weighs the risks against the benefits and hopes the end result will measure up to his or her most optimistic projections. There are risks. A surrogate mother runs the risk of having her decision backfire. If she has any doubt

about the advisability of entering into the contract, she can refuse
to sign it.

Says Hanafin, "They are not being talked into, in fact they are
being talked *out of* [surrogate arrangements]."

The surrogates are aware of the potential risks and downsides as
well as of the benefits. A few surrogate mothers have been overcome with regret and tried or wanted to keep their babies, but by
the same token, there are Wall Street investors who have jumped
out of windows because things did not turn out well.

"There is an argument made about the risk," says Andrews
"that you shouldn't do risky things with your body for money. At
the same time feminists are fighting for women to be firefighters
and in other ways put their bodies at risk, so it seems to me that
they are singling women out in terms of their reproductive function. This is the only situation they get bent out of shape about."

It is somewhat surprising that few, if any, feminists have taken
the point of view that surrogates are the most liberated of women.
It could easily be argued that surrogates are pioneers, breaking old
barriers that have long limited women's behavioral options and
their money-making potential.

Some surrogates do in fact seem to be a step ahead of everybody
else. Lisa Waters is not held back by biological destiny or anything else. "For me liberation is having a choice, and my choice
right now is to stay home and take care of my kids. But someday
I'll probably go out and start the world on fire. I can do anything."

"Official" feminists seem to be beating a retreat in comparison
to women like surrogate Kandy Harris, who is carrying on the
feminist freedom fight in the field. To her "surrogacy is a pro-
feminist thing, because it gives women the option of not having to
put their careers on hold while they have children. Go ahead, have
your career and compete with men in the marketplace. The older
you are, the harder it is to have children, but I feel women don't
have to worry about that if they can know that this option is open
to them. All is not lost."

The Remaining Confusion

Surrogates confuse us because they make us question some very
deep-seated assumptions about women. Surrogates and the women
they have babies for "are a conscience call for all other women;
they are like two sides of a folding mirror in which we see
reflected ourselves, our choices, our histories, our prejudices, our

privileges,'' says Anne Taylor Fleming in an article in the *New York Times Sunday Magazine*.[20] Surrogates who claim to be altruistic but accept money, who are independent and strong but accused of allowing themselves to be exploited, do not fit into neat categories. They seem to be full of contradictions; we cannot easily grasp what they are all about. We may understand each of their sometimes conflicting motives singly; we can't understand that these motives can coexist in the same person.

Are surrogate mothers interested in money, or are surrogate mothers altruistic?

Are surrogate mothers traditional women with traditional female values, or are they in some ways pioneers in women's liberation?

We are inclined to choose only one alternative in either question, but probably the correct answer is: all of the above.

Surrogates and surrogacy *are* confusing, and the circumstances in which these women work are not particularly pleasant. But the Baby M case has made surrogacy seem worse than it is. Public opinion on the issue of surrogacy is largely based on that tragedy, and it seems to have provoked such passions that a detached view of the practice is impossible. The Baby M case was the exception, but it has completely clouded the fact that, in general, surrogates and couples both have the best intentions and are not out to exploit each other. Where surrogacy is most likely to become nasty business is through the middleman, who does not have a personal and emotional stake in the arrangement. For the middleman babies are simply business. Agencies fulfill a necessary function, but their opportunity for exploiting both surrogates and couples is enormous. The story of their involvement is a chapter full of pleasant and unpleasant surprises.

8

The Middleman in Surrogacy

IF COUPLES ARE WELL-INTENTIONED PEOPLE DESPERATE FOR A CHILD and surrogates are eager to help them, why do they see the need to introduce a third party, the middleman, who turns an extremely personal arrangement into a business deal? Joel and Marcy know why.

Joel Mason, thirty-five, a carpenter who restored old houses in northern California, and Marcy Crane, thirty-two, a nursery school teacher, had been living together for five years when in 1981 they decided to have a child. Joel had made a girl pregnant when he was in college, and Marcy had terminated three undesired pregnancies, so they expected no problems starting a family. But after six months of trying, Marcy went to the gynecologist, who told her that she was in all likelihood sterile, probably as a result of the abortions or the IUD she had been using as birth control. However, being a modern couple, Joel and Marcy looked for modern solutions to their infertility.

Through a coworker at the nursery school, they met Dawn Keller, eighteen, who looked just like Marcy's sister and claimed to adore children. Having heard about a successful private surrogate arrangement that produced a healthy boy, Marcy approached

Dawn with the idea of her becoming pregnant by Joel. Dawn agreed with alacrity. "The vibes were right."

Keeping it all within the family, the trio decided to do the inseminations without medical assistance. For several months, visits by Joel to Dawn's apartment became part of his daily work schedule.

When Marcy began to feel left out of the creation of their baby, she wanted Dawn to move in with them, and Joel, who "was afraid she would get pregnant by somebody else," agreed. "I didn't want to take any chances," he says.

By six months later, when pregnancy was achieved, Dawn, who enjoyed all the attention lavished on her, was for all intents and purposes a member of the family.

"It was like having a grown child in the house," recalls Marcy.

But the arrangement had its advantages. Marcy could make sure that Dawn had a healthy diet and that she stayed away from drugs and alcohol. But when Dawn began to act as if she was "the real woman in the house," Joel and Marcy had her move into a small apartment.

"It was expensive, what with Dawn's rent and doctor bills," says Marcy. "We were paying about eight hundred dollars a month, more than we had counted on and more than we could really afford."

Although Marcy accompanied Dawn to doctor's appointments, the relationship changed from being "a love feast to polite formality."

Dawn was strong and healthy, but as the pregnancy progressed, she began to hate the way her body looked, and "she started to talk about how it would be after *our* baby was born. She made lists of names, names she had seen in magazines or heard on television," Marcy recalls.

Marcy got worried about the legal aspects of their situation.

"When we first made the deal with Dawn, she didn't want any money. She said that a business deal was against her spiritual beliefs," Marcy remembers. "She thought of the baby as a kind of gift to us, a love gift."

Joel believed everything would be all right once the baby was born, but Marcy insisted on seeing a lawyer. With his assistance, Dawn signed a contract in which Joel and Marcy agreed to pay all her expenses plus $2,500 "compensation for lost wages," as the lawyer put it, to make it stand up in court.

Dawn delivered a healthy girl, whom Joel and Macy named Michelle. They took the baby home and, says Marcy, "At first it seemed like finally everything was going to be the way we imagined. Michelle was a beautiful, happy baby and Dawn did not seem much interested. Dawn came by a time or two, but I didn't encourage her to visit, so we barely saw her during the first couple of weeks.''

Marcy and Joel traveled back East to introduce the baby to its grandparents. When they returned they were in for a shock.

"I think it was a combination of postpartum blues plus the influence of some people who convinced Dawn we'd taken advantage of her," says Marcy. "Two days after we got back from Delaware, Dawn shows up and tells us she can still change her mind about giving up Michelle and she is thinking about taking the baby back.''

Marcy and Joel were terrified. Their lawyer had not explained to them that it was necessary to go through a legal adoption procedure.

"We got another lawyer," says Joel, "and finally some good advice. He thought the way we'd handled the whole thing was pretty dumb, and in retrospect, I guess it was.''

After a week of negotiations, tears, promises, and vows of everlasting friendship, Dawn agreed to sign the adoption papers, but only after surreptitious payment of an additional $10,000.

"That ten grand was going to be a down payment on a bigger house. I'm not saying Michelle is not worth it, but what started out with all these high principles ended up as a cash-and-carry thing,'' says Joel. "Dawn couldn't be budged on that ten thousand–dollar price. I guess she read about it or saw it on television. For someone who never made more than minimum wage, ten thousand dollars must have seemed like an awful lot of money.''

Marcy and Joel now live in Massachusetts. They left California because they were afraid Dawn's presence could interfere with raising their daughter, now approaching her fifth birthday.

"Everybody—our friends, the people Dawn knew—everybody was aware of what had gone on. I just didn't want Michelle raised in that atmosphere,'' says Marcy, whose worst fear is that someday Dawn will appear and tell Michelle that she is her real mother. "It took a long time before I stopped worrying that somebody would come and take her away from us.''

"The one good thing about it,'' says Joel, "is that Dawn really looks like Marcy's sister, so Michelle now looks more like Marcy than like me. She looks just like the daughter we would've had together.''

Their story had a happy ending, but Marcy, Joel, and Dawn

stumbled into many problems they had not foreseen when they started out with the best of intentions.

Surrogacy arrangements are complicated—emotionally, financially, and legally. It is for this reason that surrogacy agencies have assumed the task both of warning people about the inherent problems and of minimizing problems. Agencies came into being when couples who, like Joel and Marcy, had made their own arrangements needed a lawyer to guide them through the problems they encountered, and to legalize the adoption of the child. The earliest couples to venture into surrogacy came to Noel P. Keane.

Keane, forty-eight, a lawyer in Dearborn, Michigan, and a church-going Catholic, rushed in where others feared to tread. He has become well known both nationally and as a local personality. Even the local taxi driver points out with guarded pride that Keane was the one who started it all. But, asked if he approves or disapproves of Keane's fame as the kingpin of surrogacy, the driver shrugs his shoulders, not willing to get into a discussion with a passenger who, for all he knows, could get steamed up about it. The taxi stops behind a light blue Mercedes convertible parked in front of 930 Mason Street, Noel Keane's new offices.

The first five years of his career in surrogacy Keane oversaw only five births, but business has escalated since then. His score as of this writing is 178 babies, with 30 more in the making, and an untold number in the arranging stage. He has been referred to as "a one-man baby boom."

Although it is Saturday, his elegant offices are open for business. In the corridor, surrogates are waiting with their husbands and children under framed newspaper articles of Keane's success stories. There are several articles about Shannon Boff, the first *in vitro* surrogate in the country, another first for Keane. The potential surrogates are neatly dressed, coiffed, and made up; the husbands, the minor players, are of a somewhat more nonchalant appearance. One is wearing a black T-shirt and very lived-in blue jeans. A blond surrogate is letting her husband hold their cute fourteen-month-old progeny, presumably so the squirming baby will not ruffle her attire. The child throws its plastic rattle on the floor and says, "Be, be," a vocalization only her parents understand. "She is saying baby," her mother explains, almost as if the baby understands what they are all there for.

Another, more solemn-looking couple comes in with their two children, who seem to be about four and six. They rub against their parents' legs in shyness but are quiet and well behaved. The mother smiles sweetly and reveals a set of neglected teeth.

Behind a large double door of cut glass sits a couple hoping to find the carrier of their dreams. They huddle over the conference table, their skulls almost touching, apparently discussing the game plan with great concentration. Another couple, having come all the way from Venezuela, is sequestered somewhere else in the two-story building that houses Keane and his five associates.

In a large space for the secretaries, Sandy Carter, whose turn it is to work this Saturday, greets people and offers them coffee. She gets paid extra for weekend work, she volunteers, and adds, "Noel Keane is a pretty good guy to work for." There is a computer on every desk, among other things to keep track of clients and potential surrogates. Although the atmosphere in the office is relaxed, Saturday is the busy day when it comes to surrogate arrangements.

Having made his rounds of the offices where the couples are waiting to be introduced to the surrogates, Noel Keane, dressed in a madras shirt and light blue pants, and with his feet bare in worn sandals, sits down in the gray corner sofa arrangement, ready to talk. His "throne," a large black leather chair behind his desk, is at the other end of the large, tastefully appointed office, which is more colorful and cheerful than most in the august world of the law. On one wall hangs a large picture of two children clutching dolls and pressed against a chain link fence, subliminally suggesting children looking for parents.

Noel Keane leans forward, arms resting on his knees. The big bad wolf of surrogacy does not show any teeth. This guy ought to be on the defensive. He has had enough bad publicity to be expected to bite in self-defense.

A Lansing, Michigan, lawyer, Wiley Bean, age fifty-two, is handling two damage suits on behalf of Keane surrogates and has publicly been so uncomplimentary to Keane that he is being sued for slander and libel. Although he will no longer talk about Keane's operation, he has tried to shut down Keane's surrogate practice with a court injunction. And a competitor, Harriet Blankfeld of Infertility Associates in Bethesda, Maryland, says of Keane, "People hold him up as the epitome of surrogate parenting and, believe me, he's not." She has criticized Keane for not doing any formal screening of the couples who come to him and for not requiring proof of the wife's infertility.

Keane's detractors apparently have a few things to hang their hats on. Although Keane has never met Mary Beth Whitehead or the Sterns, Baby M was nevertheless born as a result of arrangements made by his "branch office" in New York City. But that is not the only court case his name has been dragged through. "There were four," he says, "two of them are pending." And without hesitation, he goes on to explain.

A German couple sued Keane for not having given the surrogate proper instructions as to when she could have intercourse with her husband. The child they thought would be theirs turned out to be the surrogate couple's. Another lawsuit concerns a woman who claims that she was coerced into being a surrogate—although, according to Keane, "it took her six months to get pregnant"— and that she received inadequate medical treatment. The child was miscarried at five months and died immediately. Both cases were dismissed.

The two cases yet to be determined are an offshoot of the Baby M case and the still unresolved Stiver-Malahoff situation, in which surrogate Judy Stiver, who gave birth to a microencephalic child fathered by her husband, alleges that improper medical testing was done for a virus that might have caused the child's defect. Although Keane expects those cases to be dismissed, too, one is inclined to think he ought to feel a bit threatened by these fiascos and their effect on his reputation. He is not.

"I think my best attribute is that I've been open one hundred percent since day one. I know we are dealing in an area that is highly suspect because of the emotional problems, the feelings, so there is not a thing in here we won't talk about to people who have a legitimate interest."

It is hard to quarrel with that assertion. Noel Keane wrote a book, *Surrogate Mothers,* about his early days in surrogacy and spared the reader none of the dirty details. Everything—the good, the bad, and the ugly—was laid out on the printed page, including the story of the desperate couple who found their own surrogate, a woman who turned out to be a drug addict, lesbian, and extortionist.

"When I was young and starting in this area—and I think because of my Irish background—I used to blush when people would kind of zero in on me as being the baby lawyer. It was brand-new, and I didn't know where I was going or if I was doing the right thing. I don't blush anymore today. I'm absolutely sure what I'm doing. I'm helping solve infertility and I have no problem with that at all. I kind of like my position in life right now, in the area we are dealing with."

The Money Angle

Keane is making a lot of money—between $100,000 and $150,000 a year. Half of his income is from the general law practice, half from surrogacy, but Keane himself now spends 99 percent of his time working with infertile clients and leaves other matters to his associates. He is not ashamed of making money off surrogacy.

"Why are so many people opposed to me making money when anybody can do it if they have the guts to stand up and take what is coming from different directions?"

Many people resent the fact that Keane makes as much money for shuffling papers as a surrogate mother does for enduring a pregnancy, and Keane's "truckloads of money" are what is most often held against him. He is the most visible "procurer," with the highest turnover, but he has a motley crowd of colleagues.

Opening a surrogate agency requires no standard qualifications—anybody can do it—and there are no state or federal regulations governing surrogate operations. At least a dozen agencies exist around the country, and they are run by doctors, lawyers, psychologists, social workers, housewives, and former surrogate mothers. They all charge a hefty fee—usually around $10,000—for linking surrogates with baby-seeking couples.

The fee, which is generally not refundable, is paid on signing the contract. The fee covers the administrative costs of the arrangements linking couples and surrogates and of the eventual adoption procedures. It also includes the administration of expenses incurred by the surrogates and separately billed to the couples: health insurance premiums, doctors' and psychologists' fees, transportation, possible hotel accommodations for the surrogates, and a number of possible additional expenses. These costs, which are only partly predictable—a surrogate may have to travel a long way for inseminations that can go on for months before pregnancy is achieved, for example—can run into the thousands of dollars.

The couples usually take care of their own arrangements and expenses for transportation to the surrogate and their hotel accommodation. The husband has to be at hand every month to deliver semen for the insemination, which can go on and on before pregnancy is achieved.

Surrogacy is an expensive way of making babies. The total cost runs anywhere from about $25,000 to $40,000.

The cheapest agency around is probably Surrogate Motherhood, Inc., of Laurel, Maryland, which is run by a former secretary, Sharon Whiteley, who herself suffered from infertility. Her low-

volume business—fifteen births as of this writing—collects a fee
of only $6,000, and Whiteley, who claims not to be in it for the
money, has yet to make a profit. Her assistant, Julie Renz, has a
full-time job and volunteers her services to the agency. Some other
outfits, however, seem to be looking for novel and sometimes
questionable ways of shaking the money tree.

Surrogate Parenting Associates in Louisville, Kentucky, whose
brochure boasts in appalling English that it is *"the world's first
organization* to evolve for purposes of bringing together childless
couples with fertile women who are willing to assist such couples
in parenting their own biologic children,'' charges a $400 admis-
sion fee to a group meeting that provides ''the necessary information with respect to the total program and process.'' This meeting
is required before further consultation because the agency, which
''endeavored to confer with prospective natural fathers on an
individual basis,'' soon found that ''such individual consultations
were not efficient either for SPA or the prospective natural father.'' Just as in a game of poker, it costs $400 just to see.

There are other ways to squeeze out a few more pennies. It is a
practice of all surrogate agencies to hold the $10,000 payment to
the surrogate mother in an escrow account until she relinquishes
the child. Some agencies, the Hagar Institute in Kansas City and
Infertility Associates International in Maryland, for example, collect the interest on that money. Keane does not, although, he says,
''I could be earning over one hundred thousand dollars a year on
the interest; I could form a corporation and say to people that part
of the administrative cost will be that interest. I don't do that.''

Creative billing may also add to an agency's income. Even
hinting at the possibility of financial impropriety provokes Keane
slightly. When asked about the billing system, he gets up, goes to
the secretaries' office, and pulls out cost sheets to make it clear
that everything is aboveboard.

''We have a cost card on every couple, and we can show every
dollar coming in and every dollar going out.''

Says Sandy Carter, who has more hands-on experience in that
department, ''We type up an invoice and attach a copy of whatever we are billing for.''

''We requested the results of everything we wanted. We wanted
everything down pat,'' says Carmen Dubois, a Keane client. Did
she see actual proof of the cost? ''Oh yes.''

But at least one agency is more inventive, as Bob and Martha
Hansen found out.

Hansen is a teacher, and his wife is a school librarian. Mrs.

Hansen, who has two children from a previous marriage, had undergone a tubal ligation. In her new marriage she had made three unsuccessful *in vitro* attempts. Desperate for a child, they contacted an agency on the East Coast that they had learned about in *Newsweek*.

They liked what they heard from the director and signed a contract during the first visit to the office without the help of a lawyer.

"We already knew that that's what we wanted to do. It was either that or nothing," they say.

But soon the Hansens' initial satisfaction with the agency turned into unease. The bills they received from the agency never included invoices from doctors or labs; they simply showed amounts under different categories with no accompanying verification.

Say the Hansens, "The bills were pretty vague. They would bill us for a doctor's visit, for medication, and this or that, and it would just be a figure they wrote down on a piece of paper."

And there were inconsistencies. A sonogram one month was $8; the next month it was $36. On one bill, two round trips for the surrogate to the doctor were $32; next time one trip was $32.

"For tax purposes and for our information we would ask for verification, but we could never get it. They just said, 'No, you can't.' They would refuse to answer or entertain our questions, and there was nothing we could do; there was no recourse that we had," the Hansens say.

The same agency bilked another couple, Joe and Nadine Ingram, out of a more substantial amount. The agency's September 29, 1986, bill to the Ingrams shows a charge for three weeks worth of hotel accommodations for their surrogate, Katie Abrams, amounting to $1320—a totally fictitious cost, because Katie always stayed at her mother's.

The agency runs on the principle of strictest anonymity, so couples do not know their surrogate and have no way of knowing what tests, transportation, and hotel costs she may actually have incurred. Everything is handled through the agency.

Only by cracking the walls of secrecy and obtaining information about couples and surrogates and getting copies of bills do these practices become known. Because couples and surrogates do not have access to any of this evidence, they, like the Hansens, may harbor suspicions of irregularities, but they are unable to substantiate them.

Surrogate Anonymity or Contact?

Surrogate agencies differ widely on the issue of anonymity. Some, like Infertility Associates International and Surrogate Motherhood, Inc., allow no contact whatsoever between couples and surrogates. The two parties do not know each other's names or addresses. Any communication between them goes through the agency, which edits out any information that might reveal the participants' identities. Surrogate Motherhood, Inc., arrived at that policy after meetings—before the agency was formally established—with psychologists, social workers, religious people, and lawyers. Sharon Whiteley, the founder, believes that psychological studies have shown that anonymity works better all around, and in any case, "That's how the board decided to do it."

William Handel's Center for Surrogate Parenting in Los Angeles insists on an initial meeting between couple and surrogate. The Hagar Institute in Topeka, Kansas, encourages a lot of anonymous letter-writing contact and even an occasional telephone hookup but does not let the future parents meet the surrogate until the delivery of the child. Keane lets the surrogate trio work out their own arrangements, but he favors an open situation.

Many couples prefer anonymity. The Hansens chose their agency because they did not want to know the surrogate mother.

"The thing we were most drawn to was the fact that the parents-to-be and the surrogate never meet, and that, we thought, would be less stressful," the Hansens say. "We thought to ourselves, what do you do? Do you invite the birth mother to the first birthday party or do you stop after the third? We didn't know how to do that?"

Harriet Blankfeld of Infertility Associates International agrees. "You can't really say to me that somewhere along the line this couple who has this baby isn't somewhere, sometime going to want to say to the surrogate mother, 'Hey look, it's been great; you did a wonderful thing, but it is time for us to be one family, one father, one mother, one child.' How do you do that without insulting someone, stepping on toes, intimidating—or whatever you want to label it—the surrogate, who is really now technically and psychologically part of that family. I think that's where the problem arises."

"I have absolutely no predetermined rules," says Noel Keane. "These are intelligent people; it is professional couples we generally deal with, who have thought about it, and they know what they can handle and what they can't handle."

If Keane encounters a couple who insist on anonymity, he tries to change their minds.

"I say, 'That may be what you want, and it may not be what you want. I understand your apprehensions and fear that this woman is either not going to give you this child or is going to bother you after'—that's why people don't want to meet the surrogate for the most part."

He also thinks contact is better for the surrogate.

"I think that a surrogate who is doing it for other than the compensation has a need to know where the child is going, and therefore I encourage contact," Keane says. "I also don't think the infertile wife knows what she would be missing by not being part of the pregnancy, by not going to prenatal visits, by not talking to this woman, by not taking control of her baby."

Keane believes the couple will regret not meeting the surrogate, so he asks them, " 'Do me and yourself the favor and at least meet some women initially'—women who are not going to be for them—and invariably they lose that fear."

Keane worked with one couple who insisted on anonymity. He is now arranging the birth of their second child by the same surrogate. This time the couple wants to meet her.

Probably all the variations on the theme of contact make sense from one point of view or the other. Face-to-face contact allows the couple and surrogate to give each other support, enhances the altruistic aspect of surrogacy, and makes it seem less like a cold, impersonal business deal. It allows the surrogate to make up her own mind about the future parents, and vice versa, and the open personal involvement of both sides in the creation of the baby can be an invaluable emotional booster to both surrogate and parents. The danger is that the relationship established may be difficult to end—for those who want it to—after the birth.

Total anonymity never creates a relationship in the first place, so there is no trauma in ending it, but everybody lives in a state of limbo during the pregnancy, and the surrogate may forever be wondering if the baby went to the kind of home she would approve of. The biggest danger of total anonymity is, however, that a terrific amount of deceit can take place with impunity when the participants are kept totally in the dark.

Any surrogate arrangement requires both a great deal of trust and circumspection, and this is especially true with agencies that allow no contact between the parties. The Hansens' agency, for instance, sent out all the right signals. Its stationery proclaims it to be a not-for-profit operation, and its director boasts about its fine record: "I think that no matter whom you talk to, you'll hear that we have a good reputation," and as proof she offers her collaboration with two prestigious hospitals.

But appearances can be deceptive. Both couples and surrogates have to be very careful before they sign their names on the dotted line of a contract.

The Contract

Regardless of how well a contract is written, it may not stand up in court, and agencies will point that out. In the first surrogate contract dispute heard in court, the Baby M case, the contract was upheld, but the decision is being appealed. Although the Baby M case established a precedent, there is no guarantee that other jurisdictions are going to follow the same line. To insure that the agency is not held responsible for broken promises, the contract generally contains a clause absolving the agency from liability if a surrogate changes her mind.

Contracts cover more than the obligations between couples and surrogates. They also stipulate the agency's duties. Some are cleverly worded not to promise the couple anything.

Selma and Richard Corson, both lawyers, were surprised at the standard contract from an apparently reputable surrogate agency on the East Coast.

"We took the contract and read it, and we were appalled," says Selma. "It was horrible. For one thing, it never once said that the agency would do anything. It never even said it would get a surrogate, if you read it carefully. The way the money is controlled is horrible; there were no safeguards, and there was never any way to get out. My husband and I fought bitterly about the contract. He didn't want to sign it; he wanted to negotiate it, but my feeling was, you don't negotiate with this director. She told us the state's attorney general had approved it. The attorney general has not approved it. Supposedly, what he has said is that he would not prosecute her for baby-selling on the grounds of this contract."

It took Selma Corson from April to August to make her mind up about signing the contract. Her husband "washed his hands of it" but did not stop his wife.

Like most agencies, Keane's primary focus is on the couple, since their resources fuel the whole operation, and the contracts they sign "are drawn up pretty darn well to represent the couple's interests."

"We have worked on these agreements for thirteen years now," says Keane, "and we think we have it down to what is the best interest for both sides."

He offers a copy of the standard agreement.

Often couples have an outside lawyer representing them, and Keane "will tolerate some changes in the agreement—not major changes." Because the agreement has been refined over thirteen years, Keane is not eager "to reinvent the wheel."

Couples usually have a lawyer check out the contract, but even if they, like Steve Peters, a wealthy businessman, are told that the agency contract offers no protection, they may well go ahead anyway. The desire to have a child overwhelms reason in many cases.

The surrogates, too, are usually represented by a lawyer—paid for by the couple. The surrogate has to find her own lawyer, as Keane surrogate Donna Regan did.

"I had my own lawyer. I had gone to her and asked her to look the contract over. We went through everything, and she told me that they have no idea if these would be valid contracts."

Donna made a few changes in the contract. "The fee for maternity clothes and that type of thing I didn't think was sufficient to cover pregnancy, and I took out the clause about amniocentesis. I didn't see any reason for it. I had my own obstetrician/gynecologist, and if she suggested that amniocentesis was necessary, it would be different, but it was something the couple didn't know enough about to suggest to me. Wherever I wanted a change, I could change it. If they were not satisfactory to the couple, we could have started again from square one."

If Keane's surrogates cannot find their own lawyer, he will arrange for one.

"I have used an attorney in my own office who has signed an acknowledgment that he works for me," Keane explains, "but under the canons of ethics he is telling them that he is representing them in their own capacity as their lawyer." It seems a somewhat dubious situation, but, says Keane, "I can honestly tell you that he has probably a hundred times more knowledge about what it is they are dealing with than most lawyers somebody will go out and hire for a one-time shot." But using an agency-appointed lawyer can backfire.

Katie Abrams, who found herself besieged by bill collectors for doctor's services that her agency was responsible for, called the lawyer recommended to her by the agency. The lawyer had collected his fee for being present at the contract signing, but when after the birth and relinquishment of her baby she asked him for help with her problems, he said, "If you received the ten thousand dollars, you have no rights."

Katie was surprised. "I thought he was supposed to be my attorney. He as much as told me that he was not representing me. He was working for the agency."

The surrogates' contract stipulates, among other things, when their fee will be paid and what kind of compensation they will receive in case of a miscarriage. Infertility Associates International does not pay a penny unless the surrogate delivers a full-term or viable child, but most other agencies pay the surrogate something for her trouble even if the couple does not end up with a baby. The Hagar Institute, for instance, pays on a prorated basis for the number of months the surrogate was pregnant.

Keane admits that his system of compensation is not perfect.

"If the baby is miscarried from the fourth month through the ninth month, we start out with a pro-ration of five hundred to three thousand dollars. If the baby is stillborn, three thousand dollars. Criticism? Yes. Why isn't she entitled to four-ninths, five-ninths, six-ninths, etc.? It's a good idea. I can simply say it is an agreement we have entered into. Some couples can afford to pay ten thousand dollars and start over again, some cannot."

The couple's contract usually states that the surrogate will have health insurance and that the couple will pay the premium from the time inseminations start until the baby is delivered. But it also usually has a clause making the couple responsible for any bills insurance does not pay. The Gallos parents of surrogate baby Annie, felt the full weight of that stipulation.

For reasons that Lorna Gallo no longer remembers, "there was a mix-up with the health insurance. We had to pay the hospital bills. That kind of aggravated us. They came to about six thousand dollars." The total expenses for the baby came to $36,000, which for Lorna, a hairdresser, was a considerable amount of money.

Apparently, insurance can be a sticky point. The Hansens, too, had problems. They had dutifully paid the surrogate's coverage for more than nine months when, two weeks before the baby's birth, they received a registered letter from their agency informing them that the surrogate's coverage had been rescinded and they were now liable for the cost of delivering the baby. The hospital bill came to $1591.80.

The reasons for the Hansens' unpleasant surprise is known. The agency had passed the surrogates, who are contractors, off as employees and enrolled them as such in Blue Cross/Blue Shield.

When Blue Cross found out about the deceit, the policies were invalidated and the Hansens wound up victimized.

Some insurance companies do not feel that they should be required to "subsidize" surrogate agencies. Katie Abrams' insurance company refused to pay her bills under her home policy when it was alerted to her surrogate role by an article in the local newspaper describing her surrogate experiences. The couple for whom she bore the child had left the country and the agency refused to pay, so she was stuck with the bills. There was a happy outcome for Katie. After many months of discussions the insurance company was forced to pay for delivery of the baby. However, the day is likely to come when insurance agencies will specify that their family policy will not cover surrogate babies.

Agency Screening Practices

The Surrogates

Before the surrogate can start inseminations, the agency requires that she be screened. Whereas some agencies have the surrogates evaluated medically and psychologically *before* the contract is signed, Keane's does not.

"The screening is *after*, just because we are working with so many couples now and surrogates are being chosen almost as fast as they come in, if you want to know the truth. The psychological and medical counseling are done post-chosen, and all of that takes about forty-five days from the time the couples sign up with a surrogate," Keane explains.

Keane will waive all other requirements, but never the medical examination. If a surrogate is not in good health—if she suffers from venereal disease or has any problems that might make pregnancy dangerous for her—she is rejected. It is obviously in the interests of both the couple and the surrogate to have the woman who is about to embark on a pregnancy tested thoroughly in order not to endanger her or the child's health.

The medical screening of the surrogate is, however, worthless to the couple unless they see the doctor's original report. At least one agency claims to test for AIDS, chlamydia, herpes I and II, rubella—"I can give you a whole page of tests," says the director— apparently considers the physician's report classified information.

"We have our own system," she explains. "We fill in the

numbers so that it will say that a pap smear was done, and it will give the dates and the result—the same with the rest of the medical screening.''

This system leaves opportunities for improvisation. Fiona Finley, who worked for this same agency from November 1984 to August 1986, claims, "In the beginning [the director] used to *tell* everybody that all the surrogates were tested for AIDS and herpes. She didn't *do* it until somebody pinned her down in the end. They wanted to see a copy of it. We had one surrogate mother, a girl who tested positive for herpes, and the director still used her as a surrogate mother. She checked it out with the doctor's office. They said that if it's not active at the time of delivery, she can deliver vaginally, but you're still taking a chance. She wrote on the form, 'Herpes negative.' She never told the couple.''

Another situation was potentially more serious.

According to another former assistant, Rita Melrose, "There was one woman who had phlebitis. That's dangerous whether you're pregnant or not. She was the perfect candidate, a college graduate, nice looking, had had two beautiful pregnancies, great home life, her personality really effervescent, really sweet, and they were going to buy a house. We went to the insemination; the doctor suggested that she not get pregnant. The doctor went through all the things telling her that she really should not get pregnant: "You know what a danger this is. You should consider it. Why do you have to do this?' ''

Rita reported the doctor's worries to the director. "Sometimes I put my foot in my mouth," she admits. "I said it is not a good idea, and I told her what the doctor had said, and she was quite upset.''

The surrogate wanted to go through with the insemination and the director did, too, and since "the decision was entirely up to the director," the surrogate was inseminated and became pregnant. The couple knew nothing about her medical problems. Apparently, the surrogate was all right and had a baby in February 1987.

Whereas the medical testing of surrogates is pretty standard, the thoroughness of the psychological evaluation varies a great deal. Most agencies probably err on the side of caution, as they do not want another Baby M case on their conscience. For the future parents, a good psychological report is almost as important as the medical examination.

Noel Keane does not have a distinguished record in the psychological department.

In a high-volume business with no hard and fast rules, there is bound to be a problem with quality control. Shirley Williams, who many years ago considered having a baby through Keane and decided against it, was appalled by the lack of thorough screening of surrogates.

"That to me was a real concern. I don't care how well adjusted a person could be, a lot of us think we can do things we can't, and it is something that needs to be talked about."

She does admit that Keane is totally open about the program and how it is run, but she thinks that honesty does not make up for the shortcomings.

"If a doctor who operates on people does not know what the hell he's doing and people die right and left, just because he's honest doesn't make him good at what he does," she says.

Keane does screen the surrogates psychologically. He uses his own consulting psychologists for the sake of convenience. But, says Keane, if the couple is not satisfied, they can pick their own psychologist to check out the surrogate. In fact, "the couple can decide to do as much additional investigation, psychological tests, I.Q. tests as they choose." And then he adds, "Very few do more than what we do here."

Donna, a Keane surrogate, says, "I would like to see a lot more screening. I think it needs to be more intensive. Philip Parker [the Michigan psychiatrist who does Keane's psychological evaluations] is too superficial. A lot of people see him as unconcerned about why you're there, and as not being someone there to help you through. I would like to see some more actual screening done so you can alleviate the problems right from the beginning."

Admits Sandy Carter, "Dr. Parker's report is little more than a form letter most of the time, so we don't even routinely send out a copy unless the couple requests it. He rarely takes a stand on whether [the woman] can be a surrogate or not." According to Carter, he only states "that he has discussed these and these issues and he feels that she will be competent to make a decision."

Keane, though, does provide surrogates with the opportunity to get independent psychological counseling during their pregnancy.

"As a matter of fact," says Donna, "it is in your contract. They will provide you with any type of medical or psychological care that you see fit, and they will pay these expenses up to, but not exceeding, six months after the date of the delivery."

Donna took advantage of that provision, and now, together with the psychologist she saw, she is running a surrogate support group— "It's like a huge kaffeeklatsch"—that Keane's office pays for.

Although it is rarely done, Keane will consider waiving the psychological test.

"If [a couple] came to me with their sister, I don't see any need for a psychological under those circumstances, or when they come here with their own surrogate and they seem to know each other."

Next to being faulted for making too much money off surrogacy, Keane is most often criticized for his allegedly superficial psychological screening. It leaves too much responsibility with the couple, who, one often suspects, need to be saved from their own blind desires for a child. That can lead to tragedies like the Baby M case. Apparently the Sterns never bothered to check out Mary Beth Whitehead's psychological report, which contained warnings.

"I'm not sure they were warnings," Keane says. "The psychologists would say there were reasons to look beyond the initial interview, but if there were reasons to say that she shouldn't be a surrogate, the psychologist would have denied her that.

"Mary Beth Whitehead was screened for another couple before the Sterns," he continues. "The other couple were both psychologists. They had the psychological report, they interviewed Mary Beth, and they chose her. The Sterns came along and chose Mary Beth sort of on the rebound because the first man had a low sperm count and couldn't get her pregnant. The Sterns probably said to themselves—I don't know this; I'm guessing—that the other couple chose her, they had her screened. They had liked what they saw in Mary Beth, so the Sterns used her, too, without ever asking for the psychological report which was available to them."

Some of Keane's failures have been monumental and have been plastered all over the front pages of the daily newspapers, but he cannot be accused of the kind of deceit practiced by another agency. The director of that agency, who has on occasion criticized Keane's minimal screening procedures, claims that in her agency the couple gets a full report and receives "the copy that comes from the psychologist. We take out the name and address and that's all . . . because we work with the concept of anonymity. They get to see the good, the bad, and the ugly, believe me, because there is no such thing as a perfect psychological on anybody."

No, but there is always room for improvement.

The assistants in this agency's office are instructed to take out anything that is uncomplimentary—some of it not very serious—and rewrite the report.

Says Rita, who worked there as an assistant, "The couple never did see the original psychological report. They saw the one that was written in the office by me or whoever was working there. Some things were taken out, naturally, that didn't sound good.''

The editorial emendations were quite successful. "They all come out looking like Mary Poppins,'' says another former assistant, Sandra King, who worked for the agency from August to December 1986.

"We asked to see the original reports,'' says Selma Corson, "and we were told we couldn't. I think they leave in things that they wish to highlight and leave out things they don't want you to see.''

The agency often has a shortage of surrogates, and with hungry couples barking at the door, the psychological evaluation may be too time-consuming.

One time, according to Fiona, a surrogate was not screened psychologically at all.

"There was this one surrogate, real cute, nineteen years old, not married, with a baby. [The director] didn't do a psychological on her or anything. She wrote the whole thing up on her, sent it out to the couple; they liked her and they accepted her. It ended up that the surrogate took off for somewhere and never showed up. They never did any inseminations or anything. [The director] made up this lie that she was going back to live with her parents. That was the end of that. Then they got another surrogate.''

This kind of psychological fiction writing is only possible in a climate of total anonymity, although that does not mean that other agencies operating with a no-contact policy see the need to withhold original reports.

Most agencies not only screen the surrogates but the future parents as well. The father-to-be is required to submit to an AIDS antibody test and give proof that he is not afflicted with any venereal diseases. Some agencies also demand to see the results of a sperm count.

Keane requires no proof of male fertility.

"Most couples before they plunk down twenty-five thousand dollars know whether the semen is viable or not,'' says Sandy Carter, Keane's assistant, and adds, "They don't have to show us proof, but without it they can't really do this,'' implying, "How could anybody be so stupid enough to come here without having been tested first?''

One agency, which makes a big to-do about its stringent medical evaluations of the father, nevertheless accepted a man and his nonrefundable $10,000, knowing that he had a low sperm count.

Some surrogate programs will not enroll a couple unless the wife has been certified as infertile by a physician. They want to eliminate people who want surrogate babies simply for the sake of convenience. Keane requires no such proof. But would he knowingly make arrangements for a couple if the wife could have her own children?

"I have never been confronted with that, but if a couple came to me and said, 'Hey, we are too busy . . .' " Keane thinks for a second. "It is hard for me to say sitting here. I could certainly say no, I would never do that—so you can write it down—but I don't know if that is true or not. If a couple came to me with some reason why, I would certainly listen to them. I don't think many women would give up the experience of carrying their own children either."

Like the Hagar Institute, Noel Keane works with single men, although not with homosexuals.

"Frankly, I don't have a problem with homosexuals," he says. "There was a couple, two men, who came to see me who were super nice guys. I liked them, but my support group and the office staff and my wife didn't think it would be a good idea. They are always talking in the abstract rather than about individuals. I'm the individualist, but we chose not to get into it in any case."

Choosing a Surrogate Partner

The crucial thing in a surrogate arrangement—for both couples and surrogates—is choosing the right "partner." All couples, of course, prefer good-looking and intelligent surrogates with a nice personality who resemble the wife as closely as possible. All surrogates are concerned that the baby they give birth to will have nice parents and a good home.

How Are They Found?

A lot of potential surrogates hear about agencies through the media. Noel Keane and Infertility Associates International get enough self-motivated women through free publicity—articles about the agencies in the news media, appearances on television, etc. During the first years of surrogacy, it was the only way to attract candidates because newpapers refused to accept ads calling for surrogates.

In the earliest days of surrogacy, Noel Keane called the now defunct *Washington Star* to place an ad in the paper calling for surrogate mothers. The newspaper's lawyers were baffled. They had never heard of such a thing and did not know what it implied but decided to find out about it. They called the attorney general's office in Michigan, from where Keane was operating, to find out if there were any laws prohibiting the practice. A search through the law books yielded no laws directly relating to surrogacy and none that outlawed it. Nevertheless the *Star* turned down the ad. "It just felt odd," said former *Star* lawyer Walter Diercks. "We didn't really know what we were getting into."

Agencies that receive less media coverage, such as the Hagar Institute and Surrogate Motherhood, Inc., rely heavily on newspaper advertising. Many of the women who respond to the ads are not suitable. Says Julie Renz of Surrogate Motherhood, Inc., "We have definitely had some doozies. It just happened with our last advertising. One was in the middle of some emotional turmoil and was doing this to strike out at a boyfriend who had dumped her after four years. She hated all men and started to cry on the phone. Another one told me that she did drugs quite frequently—PCP and a little cocaine. Not the types of person we need in this program. We also get people who sound very well educated and very determined. I always spend half an hour with them on the phone" before application forms are sent out.

The Hagar Institute, which puts "newspaper ads in all kinds of little papers in Kansas," rejects one out of every seventeen callers on the spot. The Center for Surrogate Parenting in Los Angeles, which gets surrogate applicants through the media and advertising as well as through referrals from physicians, interviews only 50 percent of those women who offer their services. Those who make it past the initial interview are then screened before their files are passed on to the couples.

What Qualifications Are Required?

Some surrogate applicants are rejected for not so obvious reasons. Many agencies will only accept surrogates who have already had children of their own. They agree with Steve Peters, who is hoping to get his surrogate pregnant: "Doing this with a rookie who has never had the experience of having a baby and not knowing what it felt like when it was born I think would be suicidal."

Although there have been occasional exceptions, Surrogate Motherhood, Inc., according to its lawyer, will not even accept women who express a desire to have more children of their own later, as that kind of woman might be tempted to keep the surrogate baby.

Infertility Associates International demands a minimum of a high school diploma; the Center for Surrogate Parenting cannot use women who do not have a drivers license, apparently a necessary tool of survival in the Los Angeles area.

Some agencies prefer local women. Others will accept them from all over the country and fly them in, a practice that adds to the cost.

Selecting the mother of your child is a rather awe-inspiring undertaking. "There is no decision in the world that I can think of that's more important," says Selma Corson, and yet it is frequently done on the basis of relatively flimsy information. This is especially true where anonymity is the rule and no checking on the information is possible.

In Noel Keane's outfit, couples can check on surrogates as much and as long as they want. In his New York office, couples start by going through a loose-leaf binder containing profiles of "probably a hundred women available," says Steve, who was considering arranging for a surrogate baby through Keane. "I liked the information supplied on the surrogates. The basic data sheet contained information about age, the number of children already born to the surrogate, family history, whether their grandparents were still alive, national origin, height, weight, and photos. There was also a written questionnaire, where the surrogate had filled out questions like 'Why do you want to become a surrogate?' 'Do you think you'll have problems giving up the child?' It is a very revealing document that gave you information about both what their philosophies were and how intelligent they were."

In Keane's Michigan office, couples and surrogates get what they see. They meet each other and can ask each other questions before deciding to collaborate on their unusual venture.

Bad Experiences with Surrogacy Agencies

Where anonymity reigns, both couples and surrogates have to rely on the psychological reports forwarded by the agency and the photographs attached to the surrogate's file.

In most cases, the agency sends out several files for the couples to choose from, but one program forwards only one at a time because, according to the director, "there is no fair in comparing." Usually, she says, the couples do not go beyond two profiles before deciding. If they are not satisfied at the point, she asks them, "Why don't you want those surrogates?" If the reply is, for example, "They are too short," she responds, "Well, I'm sorry, I don't have anybody six feet tall." The director claims that the quality of her surrogates is so good that if a couple has not chosen at that point "their expectations for a surrogate mother are simply unrealistic."

Selma Corson had a different and perhaps unique experience of the agency's selection procedures.

"We signed the contract, and we kept calling for files," she recounts. "[The director] never phoned, never returned calls. Finally one day she called and said, 'I have a wonderful surrogate for you. She was scheduled to be the surrogate for somebody else, but she turned them down, and she was scheduled for artificial insemination on Sunday.' This was Thursday, and we had to decide by Sunday."

When the Corsons had talked to the agency initially, they had been shown three sample surrogate files but had been told then that the women were not available, as they had already been chosen. The Corsons remembered them well because they had liked their profiles. The surrogate described on the phone sounded very familiar to Selma.

"That's the woman you showed us in April who wasn't available," she said.

"Oh no," demurred the director, "it couldn't be."

"I know it is the woman you showed us in April," Selma insisted.

"Oh well," parried the director, "she is very fussy; she has turned down other people."

"What makes you so sure she won't turn us down," Selma asked.

"You're just perfect," the director reassured her. "She turned one couple down because the father was too old."

Selma admits to being foolish. "Of course, wanting to believe everything she said and thinking this was a pretty good surrogate, we took the file home and made the decision in one day."

The Corsons did find it odd that the agency had not given them any files for weeks, and then suddenly they had to decide immediately because the inseminations were already scheduled. Selma suspects that another couple had backed out because the surrogate did not get pregnant, and that the surrogate was never told about the switch of fathers. The surrogate did not get pregnant by Richard Corson.

Apparently, this agency, which will switch fathers on a surrogate, has also switched surrogates on couples who have agonized over the choice of the mother. According to Rita, "[The director] has been known to switch surrogates without telling the couple because perhaps the surrogate could not continue or something happened." The director insists that "even though each of the surrogates is different, they are basically the same," but it is doubtful that the couples would share her opinion.

Getting a surrogate pregnant is not always easy. Sometimes nature is recalcitrant, and sometimes surrogates do not show up for their scheduled inseminations, three each cycle.

Fiona remembers those difficult situations.

"There were cases where the surrogate would not turn up for an insemination. The father would never be told, the specimen would just be dumped. One surrogate didn't show up for all three of them, and the father came flying in from Florida. [The director] knew on the first day that the surrogate wasn't going to show for the next two. She still had him go to the doctor's office each day and had him pay for his hotel and everything. She never told him, called him up the next month: 'Your surrogate got her period.' "

If six months or more go by without conception, the couple can choose a new surrogate. But there is a little money to be made on a surrogate who does not conceive. This is how it works. After six months of no pregnancy, the surrogate is passed on to a new couple, who will then try for another six months, and so on and so on, and all the couples are charged $300–400 for the psychological and medical screening of the surrogate, who is only tested once.

King claims that "there was one surrogate who was used three times by three different couples." The Corsons were probably caught in that merry-go-round.

Then there is the opposite story, the surrogate who is already pregnant when the inseminations start.

Finley recalls that one couple had had two surrogates—one did not show up for inseminations, the other one got sick—before they were given a third one who had already conceived. "It ended up that this girl was already pregnant. She delivered a month or two months before her due date. She never had a pregnancy test before all the inseminations. None of them ever did. I'm sure they do now."

King remembers the surrogate. She "delivered in late January.

What no one had seen was that her physician had moved up the due date by six weeks. In other words, this woman was artificially inseminated when she was already pregnant by somebody else, or it was the largest premature baby ever born—one for the *Guinness Book of Records*. I don't know how the agency got away with that one.''

The Corsons ended up dropping out of the program. Their first surrogate did not get pregnant and was suddenly withdrawn. The next surrogate they were offered turned them down, and the subsequent one was the last straw for Selma.

''The woman was on birth control pills,'' Selma explains, ''and the medical note said she would go off them and therefore was ready for inseminations. It also talked about her temperature charting of her ovulation, which is absolutely ridiculous, because you don't ovulate when you're on the pill. First we get a surrogate who is supposedly infertile, and now we are offered one who is not off the pill yet. You don't ovulate for a number of months, and you should not try to get pregnant for at least six months after you go off the pill, and here [the director] is scheduling inseminations for a month later.''

The agency, which for some reason declares that it will never use the same surrogate twice, nevertheless does. The surrogate the Corsons rejected was a repeater, who conceived immediately the first time around. She became a surrogate for the second time. After the Corsons rejected her, she was assigned to somebody else. She has yet to conceive—after seven months of inseminations.

The Corsons got the money for the surrogate's fee back after many phone calls, but Selma was furious to see that it was drawn on the director's own account. Selma had originally insisted that it be put in an escrow account and not be commingled with agency funds, which in the event of bankruptcy are subject to creditors. Selma hopes to retrieve at least part of the fee paid to the agency and is considering a lawsuit.

Just as it is important for the couple to get reliable information on the surrogate, surrogates want to know or at least get a feeling of what the future parents are like. The parties meet each other; they can judge for themselves. Where they do not, they have to trust the agency's information.

Katie Abrams signed up with an agency and chose to have a baby for an American couple where the husband was ''a country doctor who made house calls.'' Katie liked that, and through the agency she had a little correspondence with the couple, who came across to her ''as nice and sensitive.'' Everything went fine. Katie got pregnant and was such a good surrogate that the director of the agency wanted to show her off to the press. She delivered the baby by an unexpected cesarean section and relinquished the baby as agreed.

It was not until after the delivery that something started to nag at Katie. After the delivery she found out in a round-about way that the father was indeed a doctor, but "well, what country did he practice medicine in?" It turned out that the couple was Israeli. That in and of itself did not bother Katie, but the fact that she had not been told the truth did. She became almost paranoid with fear that nothing she had been told was "on the up and up."

"The first thought that ran through my mind was that the baby was going to be sold on the black market; and all I could think about was, 'How am I ever going to justify within myself what I have done?' "

Katie is now assured that the baby was adopted legally, but although she signed the final papers in November 1986, as of the end of June 1987 she had still not received her copy of the adoption papers. No matter how many times she calls the agency, the papers do not arrive. Because of her lingering unease, Katie would dearly love to get a sign from the parents that everything is all right. Since the delivery, she has never heard a word from them, in spite of the fact that she has sent them several letters through the agency. Katie does not know if the couple ever received her letters but is becoming suspicious that both her letters to the couple and perhaps a thank-you note from them to her have been "trash-canned."

Says Fiona Finley, "[The director] withholds letters. As soon as the surrogates have delivered, she doesn't want to hear from them again."

That was also true, says Rita Melrose, when she worked for the agency. "Once the surrogates have that check, nothing else is said. They go home, and she doesn't want to hear from them again. She doesn't want to hear about any problems they have. They have gone through their contract, they have abided by it, and she supposedly has abided by hers, and that's it."

The Need for Regulation

Most surrogate agencies, while not shunning the income, are in the business to perform a service. But there are enough examples of grossly unethical behavior in the surrogate business to make outside intervention absolutely necessary. One way to avoid all the problems is, of course, to outlaw the practice of surrogacy altogether, and that is what Keane critic Wiley Bean wants to do.

"It is irrelevant what I feel about the mechanics about a particular operation, whether program A has resulted in more lawsuits than program B. If, for example, Noel Keane had a heart attack and could no longer be in business, would that stop what is going on in this field? The answer is no."

To Bean it is not a question of introducing laws and regulations, because the problems are inherent in the practice of surrogacy. Assuming the worst, he asks rhetorically, "Does the surrogate mother have the right to take the risk? Can she sell her child for money and leave her husband and children without a mother? At what point do we say, 'It is your duty to your husband and children not to take a life-threatening risk and leave them behind for the sake of money?' "

Other voices call for the elimination of agencies, wanting to make surrogacy a private matter. Keane for obvious and not so obvious reasons does not think that is a good idea.

"The legislation they are trying to pass now is to do away with the middleman's responsibility. The craziest thing they could ever do is to do away with somebody who has total accountability to some professional organization," Keane argues. "I have full accountability to the bar association. If I do one thing out of line, I have to account to the bar association immediately."

Keane, being a lawyer, may not need a lot of policing, but there are surrogate entrepreneurs who have no accountability to anybody and who can do whatever they please.

Of all the agencies operating in this country, only one, the Hagar Institute, is licensed. The state of Kansas granted it a license as a child placement agency because it is run on the same principles as an adoption agency. Its founder and director, Beth Bacon, sees its status as "an indication of the growing acceptance of surrogate motherhood." She actively sought the license and welcomes, she says, the visits from inspectors.

"They come every year and look at everything. It is a help to us. They deal with evaluations and child placement all the time and they have good input."

Surrogate Motherhood, Inc., keeps their state attorney general's office informed of the agency's business on an entirely voluntary basis, because Whiteley, the founder, believes that her program could be a model to consider when future legislation is introduced.

Legislation is badly needed, but until regulations are in place, it is up to the couples and surrogates themselves to watch out for abuses before they sign on. Unfortunately, neither is likely to take a cool look at the situation. Surrogates often approach an agency too full of idealism and eagerness to help an infertile couple to be objective.

Says Katie, who had a bad experience, "My intentions were so good. To think that I've been involved in something that wasn't on the up and up . . . The idea of it broke my heart."

Selma Corson, who is angry about her experience, admits that as a lawyer she ought to have known better. But, she says, it is hard to convey "how desperate you are when you walk in. You don't do all the things you would normally do in a transaction of this size and nature, because you want to believe that everything is okay. You see all the inconsistencies, and you keep pushing them under the rug. Things are so obviously wrong, and you just close your eyes to them. That's the sad part."

There are agencies operating on the principle of total anonymity that are perfectly honest, but total anonymity gives an agency an enormous amount of power and an unusual opportunity to exploit people who are extremely vulnerable.

"We were told so many things in the initial meeting which turned out not to be true," the Hansens say. "If we knew before what we know now, it would be a different story." They are, in spite of everything, happy to have a healthy baby. "We didn't want to know the mother. Now we have changed our minds. We realized at the end there was nothing we could do because it was all anonymous and therefore the agency could make it anything it wanted to."

There is no such thing as a perfect surrogacy agency, and all of them should be approached with caution and skepticism. The most telling indications of a decent agency are openness as far as it is possible and adherence to standard business procedures.

9

The Moral and Ethical Issues of New Reproductive Technologies

IN ROOM 2203 OF THE RAYBURN HOUSE OFFICE BUILDING IN Washington, D.C., a group of middle-aged men and one older woman, seated at a half-circle wooden desk with pitchers of ice water, peer over their bifocals at the testifying scientists.

Standing room only.

No one jumps to hear such matter-of-fact talk of egg and sperm, of $50 semen counts, of cervical mucus and urine hormone kits, but some squirm uncomfortably, wishing they did not have to think about such things. Is this what politics has come to?

Men and women on Capitol Hill hurriedly stuff folders of information for the press. A woman in a navy blue dress with a laminated Capitol Hill identification card around her neck, holds a diaper in her hand while her mother looks worriedly at the baby in the baby carriage.

"She's hungry," the grandmother says. "She's chewing her fingers. What are you going to do?"

"Wait till she cries," says the professional mother, nervously eyeing her boss, a congressman.

"Today, the Select Committee on Children, Youth and Families will examine the current and emerging reproductive treatments," announces Congressman George Miller, "and explore the complex medical, legal, and ethical questions these methods pose for our society, as well as our children and families." In some cases, the congressman from California notes, the technology has "surpassed society's ability to assimilate it, forcing us to confront some very basic, very delicate questions," which "demand future enlightened consideration."

Whether the debates are "enlightened consideration" or justifications of threatened belief systems, at least the people gathered here have expended considerable thought on the theme—reproduction. As one conservative thinker tells the politicians, "Sexual intercourse without babies has been followed by babies without intercourse," and babies without sexual intercourse is what these politicians address.

Two panels of experts have been called to testify.

Panel 1 consists of two clean-cut looking male doctors—the scientific director of an *in vitro* fertilization clinic, Gary Hodgen, and an endocrinologist from George Washington University, Robert Stillman—a young female doctor with an earnest smile from the Bureau of Maternity in New York City, Wendy Chavkin; and a worried priest, Richard Doerflinger, from the National Conference of Bishops.

Panel 2 consists of a hyper young law professor at the University of Texas, John Robertson, speaking adamantly for "procreative liberty"; a health law professor from Boston University, George Annas; an attractive blond research fellow from the American Bar Foundation, Lori Andrews; and the director of a conservative think tank in Virginia, Robert Marshall.

These are the people the television talk shows call when the subject of alternative reproduction comes up.

Each is like an informal political action committee representing some segment of the world they believe to be victimized either by putting reproductive technologies into forward or reverse gear.

Victims: The infertile. "One in every five or six couples, or fifteen to twenty percent of the married," notes Dr. Stillman. "That amounts to millions and millions of American couples involuntarily denied the fundamental biological right of procreation and having a family."

Victims: Unborn children. "I was especially pleased to be invited to testify," says George Annas, "because I believe the public debate over these issues [has] . . . almost no consideration of the best interests of the resulting children."

Victims: the adopted. "Why are we taking for granted the

pursuit of a genetically related child in the face of so many children without parents?'' asks Wendy Chavkin.

"We approve of adoption," says the priest, Mr. Doerflinger, "but not of the surrogate situation."

"Let me get this clear, Mr. Doerflinger," says Congressman Morrison, "and I have a special interest in this because I'm adopted. Are you saying that a child is less loved if it's not a biological child?"

"No, I didn't say that."

"Well, it seems to me that surrogacy is very close to adoption," observes Morrison. "It seems to me, with your argument of biological precedence, a surrogacy situation would be preferable . . ."

"It's very complicated," replies Doerflinger, "But the implications for baby-selling are there; I don't think it's good public policy."

Says Congressman Ted Weiss, a senior congressman who has sat quietly through the debates, "We had yuppies, now we have TINCs—you've heard of those—two income, no children. Well, now these people have changed their minds, now they want children. And they want them badly. I was talking to a woman who had a child and wasn't married, and I saw her sometime later and she had a wedding ring on, and I said, 'Did you get married?' She said, 'No, I had to buy a wedding ring because people on the subway were offering me up to thirty-five thousand dollars for my child. These are people with resources and they are going to find a child."

Congressmen have convened and experts have testified on what used to be a private matter, discussed not in a congressional hearing room but in the bedroom of private citizens. They are discussing how people should or should not have children.

As long as people have babies through normal intercourse, there is not much any outsider can say about it—the right to procreate, or at least to attempt it, has rarely been questioned. But there are a growing number of people for whom intercourse will not do the trick, and they have to resort to alternative means of reproduction. These alternatives include everything from artificial insemination by donor, *in vitro* fertilization, and egg and embryo transfers to the use of surrogate mothers. The one thing that all the different "treatments" have in common is their removal from the bedroom and the involvement of third parties. In some cases impregnation is anything but private, featuring not only sophisticated electronic devices but a cast of doctors, nurses, and medical students, with television monitors narrow-casting the proceedings to visitors in the gallery. Nevertheless infertile couples, for whose benefit the show must go on, will still insist that their decision to have a baby is a private matter and that they, like other Americans, are justified in exercising their right to have children.

John Robertson, a law professor at the University of Texas, one of the panelists at the hearing on Capitol Hill, and generally recognized as the most prominent spokesman for "procreative liberty" would agree: ". . . procreation by fertile or infertile married couples is a constitutionally protected right, subject to state limitation only for compelling reasons and not merely to express distaste or moral condemnation of an alternative style of reproduction. . . . Surely infertile couples should have the same right to rear children that are biologically or gestationally related to one or both of them that fertile couples do, if the means for creating such children exist."[1]

Not so, says Sidney Callahan, associate professor of psychology at Mercy College, Dobbs Ferry, New York. "The claim that an individual's right to reproduce would be violated if fertility teatments are not available to any individual who requests them seems wrongheaded. The right to marry, for example (itself not absolute), does not obligate society to provide spouses."[2]

As in all debates that involve the Constitution, it is the balance between individual rights and the rights of the state that are being weighed.

"Some persons will see benefits to a single individual or couple as dominant. Others will view potential risks to society as a whole as taking precedence over individual benefits," writes the American Fertility Society in a ninety-four-page examination of ethical considerations of the new reproductive technologies. "Applying the person criterion, one must take into account that the human person is both individual and social."[3]

When it comes to infertility, there is a potential conflict between the individual and society. Society as a whole does not really need any more children than those who come naturally, but for the couple who wants a child they cannot conceive, infertility is a devastating tragedy. Childless people will often go to lengths that may not only seem crazy but selfish to people who have babies without the help of medical science.

John Layton, a forty-two-year-old lawyer in Cape Girardeau, Missouri, believes the inability of infertile people to accept their lot has something to do with "the me generation." "People began to say, 'I come first,' and began to think about themselves to the exclusion of others. People used to view themselves within the context of their family and friends, but now it is 'I come first.' If you justify the idea that I'm entitled to have things my way, then there is no limit, regardless of the effect it may have on others."

Finding the right balance in the future may be increasingly difficult as more barren people and their doctors forge ahead with new and exotic ways of coaxing children into the world. They set the pace, and the policy makers can only try to keep up. Meanwhile the public worries about the destination.

Wanted Children, Wanted Parents

"Sometimes I walk out of those sessions saying, 'Wouldn't it be better if this couple didn't have a child?' " observes Susan Mikesell, who counsels infertile couples at Washington, D.C.'s, Columbia Hospital for Women before they embark on the *in vitro* venture. But "knowing I can't do anything about it, I never say that, because everybody has a right to have children."

The new ways of making babies have broken the constraints of the biological family, and they have allowed tightly held concepts to be divided that were never divided before. They all separate sex from procreation, DI and surrogacy separate child-begetting from childrearing, and all of them remove conception from the bedroom. Traditionally, biology has kept all these things together and given society a semblance of reproductive order.

It was the advent of contraception that began to pull these things apart. The control of human procreation started with the introduction of devices that blocked the flow of sperm to egg—technically simple, but socially and morally hard to accept. The debate over this radical concept raged—much like the public discussion of reproductive technologies today—on all levels of society. Would it eliminate the undesirable elements of society? Would it lead to social depravation? Was it a health hazard? Was it economically reasonable? Regardless of the opinions held, everybody could agree with the famous newpaper pundit Walter Lippman that ". . . whether or not birth control is eugenic, hygienic and economic, it is the most revolutionary practice in the history of sexual mores."[4]

Thanks to the now almost century-old campaign for birth control, which has run on the moral premise that all children should be wanted children, today fertile Americans who want to avoid bearing offspring have all the technical and legal means to do so.

The right to bear only wanted children is considered by many Americans to be a basic human right. Excepting abortion, most of us no longer worry about the ethics of creating only wanted children; we now debate the issue of creating children for those who want them.

The new birth methods bring very wanted children into the world. They also bring up the question of whom society considers desirable parents.

Unlike people who adopt, couples who seek babies by the help of medical technology or through surrogate agencies do not usually have to prove their fitness as parents. In principle, anyone whose body responds to the "cure" and who has the money to pay for it can have a baby. That is a leap with social consequences, made possible not only by the new methods of conception but by a changing social climate. The novel ways of making babies are both the result and the cause of rapid social change.

By the time the first test tube baby was born and the first few surrogate babies squirmed in their cribs, feminists had already left home and joined the workplace; the average age of pregnancy had risen and lifestyles ran the gamut from "trial marriages" (more accurately described as living together) to single parents, even to gay parents.

Both the insides and outsides of marriage had changed. According to various surveys, in 1979 two-thirds of never-married women had had intercourse by the time they were nineteen. From June 1979 to June 1980, there were 1,184,000 divorces in the United States. There were 1.2 million children under the age of eighteen whose parents had divorced in 1978, which amounts to 18.1 children under the age of eighteen per 1,000 members of the population, a rate that is three times that typical of the 1950s. Estimates of children living in single-parent homes in 1980 vary from 11 million to 17 million.

"We are living in an age where many adults find it difficult to make lasting commitments to each other, but still consider having and raising children to be meaningful," says Dr. Susan Robinson.[5]

Apparently, just as orgasm, the big O, was the end point of the sexual revolution, a child of one's own became the end goal of the goal-driven generation of the 1980s, who appear almost obsessed with children.

Single Parents and Reproductive Technologies

The belief that love, marriage, and children are all part of the same social package was already rather shaky, when singles began to demand to have children by means intended and created to relieve infertility among the married.

"I always assumed I would get married and have kids, somewhere between two and four," says Linda Olson, a forty-two-year-old Ph.D. scientist working at the National Institutes of Health. "I never thought that my career would be more important than having kids, but as I approached thirty, I realized that it wasn't a guaranteed thing."

Linda had a problem—no husband.

"There were a number of single women in my situation who wanted to get married but found the numbers were not in their favor," she says. "Also, highly educated women discovered that men were not brought up to be comfortable dealing with highly educated women. I waited till I was thirty-five and tried every single activity in the book. I wanted a family, and it wasn't that I wanted to do it on my own."

Even as her biological clock ticked away, she was patient, but at age thirty-eight, after having picked up the emotional pieces of an unsuccessful relationship, she decided, "Okay, nothing is going to stop me now. Now is the time to go and get pregnant."

Thanks to donor insemination, Linda became the mother of twins at age forty-two—after several miscarriages.

Ever since donor insemination became available for single women of any sexual persuasion, they have been able to have children without the socially required man in their lives.

"DI has a tremendous potential for expanding the options women have in their lives," says Francie Hornstein, originator of a DI program at the Los Angeles Feminist Women's Health Center. "I think a lot of people get married solely because they want to have children. And maybe now those people—mostly women—won't feel that they have to get married."[6]

Among the 1,000 members nationwide of "Single Women by Choice," some have used donor insemination. These modern day Hester Prynnes are not wearing scarlet letters. The term *illegitimate* has little meaning for women whose biological clocks are chiming the eleventh hour. These women in their late thirties and early forties, who came of age in the sixties and worked for and benefited from feminism, are reaping their final reward from a society that doesn't frown on much of anything they do anymore.

Although "the data really does not exist," Dr. Jerome Sherman, director of the AATB, says that there is increasing interest in using sperm banks by single women. At the Sperm Bank of Northern California, a bank that was created in part to meet the needs of single women and lesbians, the mean age of recipients is thirty-six and the largest age group in 1983—152 women—was of women aged thirty-five to thirty-nine years old. Sixty-four percent were in or had completed graduate school, 60 percent were unmarried, and 11 percent divorced.[7] At Idant, too, a growing number of single women are taking matters of childbearing into their own hands. The customers are both heterosexual and gay.

The single woman has traditionally been an awkward member of society—an odd fit at dinner parties, a threat to married women, and an unproductive member of society as a result of her refusal to reproduce legitimately within the confines of marriage. "In no society anywhere has there been a warm and accepting home for the unmarried," notes Luther Baker . . . "The situation has been especially serious for the single female. . . . Set in a society which idolizes motherhood and views the purpose and function of the female sex as biological progeneration, these 'unhappy misfits' are often considered by the community as a whole, and even by themselves, as a kind of vague neuter gender . . . left just outside the pale of full human acceptance."[8]

Many single women who have for years lamented their lowly status as singles are now asserting their right to be fruitful and multiply, too. In another age, their children would have been labeled bastards.

For many years there was great reluctance on the part of physicians to allow DI for single women. Declared one medical association in 1962, "Artificial insemination of an unmarried woman is in conflict with the social order, and inadmissible on medical ethical grounds."[9]

One physician, mulling over the "problematic" situation of whether or not he should inseminate single women, noted, "Basically [I] try and put the decision off . . . say there are no donors. If she's older, say thirty, okay, but not the younger ones, not twenty-one and not a lesbian."[10]

Another doctor developed a typology.

"Basically there's three kinds of single women. There's the activists, the lesbians that are single by choice. They are feminists, they don't like the establishment. They come in here and demand sperm and don't want their ovulation controlled. Then there's the emotionally ill ones . . . basically I get them therapy and their interest in DI disappears. Then there's the healthy, normal, well-adjusted single women whom life just has not seen fit to provide with a partner. I inseminate these single women . . . but, I still feel a bit uncomfortable about it . . . but, I do it. I've come to terms with that. . . ."[11]

Even if doctors don't relish the idea of choosing who are to be parents, they are placed in that position by women who see no other way to accomplish what up to now has required marriage.

"Social evolution happens in society because of a felt need," says psychotherapist Fae Pannor, founder of the Alternative Parenting Network in Los Angeles, which helps many single women become parents. "They wouldn't be doing it unless there was a deep need. Nobody comes along and suggests that they do this. The reality is that it's what people are doing and we're going to have to find ways to make it [psychologically] healthy.

"Men have been in control of this for hundreds of years," says Ponnor. "They've left babies left and right and they couldn't have cared less. Now women are taking control."

The movement for making DI available to single woman is a direct outgrowth of the women's movement, which showed that women could be independent. It is also a direct outgrowth of the sexual revolution, which pushed the idea that sex was less for making babies and more for pleasure. The new intentionally single mothers take their sex for pleasure and relegate the conception process to another area of life. It is not so much technology as rampant social changes that have made single women see the potential in artificial insemination.

"It took me years to realize that being a lesbian and being a mother were not two mutually exclusive concepts," says one single mother. "However, I had no desire to have sex with a man just for the purpose of becoming a parent. There are risks like getting a venereal disease or meeting Mr. Goodbar—you know, someone who could get violent—and there is the emotional problem of having sex with somebody you do not love. I didn't want to have a baby under those circumstances, but I very much wanted to be a mother. . . . for me, things turned out as I had hoped. I have a family, and my career, and did not have to have sex with a man I did not love to make it happen."[12]

Men, who generally enjoy life-long fertility, have always been seen as having more options. When Linda Olson was considering donor insemination, an older, unmarried male coworker was the only person who conveyed his negative reaction.

"He had always seen his situation as having more flexibility," says Linda. "He could contribute his part to a pregnancy well into his fifties, and I was worrying about whether I would be fertile at thirty-nine or forty. When I told him what I was going to do, it was something that a guy in his situation could not do, and I think that was part of the reason for his negativism."

"The ticking of our biological clocks has made us face the fact that we could no longer wait for marriage before starting our families," reads the Single Women by Choice brochure. "Some of us accidentally became pregnant and discovered we were thrilled. Some of us intentionally conceived with a man. Others went to a doctor for artificial insemination or found a child we could adopt. Most of us would have preferred to have brought a child into a good marriage. However, while we have a lifetime to marry, nature is not so generous in allotting childbearing years."[13]

"It wasn't that hard of a decision," says Jamie, about her quick decision to be a parent. "Being in private practice, I have a lot of flexibility and a good income. I had done everything in the world I wanted to do *except* get married and have children."

In many states there is considerable uncertainty about the legal rights and duties of all parties involved, including the mother, offspring, physician, and donor. Things are particularly confused for single mothers. Who is the legal father? Does the biological father, if he wants, have visitation rights? Can the offspring sue the physician for "wrongful life" in case he or she is abandoned, abused, or otherwise neglected by his or her mother? DI laws are confused enough for married women, but doubly so for single women.

But the new technologies and the detachment they allow us may be in danger of deluding us about the superfluity of men.

"There is no such thing as a fatherless family," notes psychologist Rona Achilles. "It still takes a sperm and egg, at least for now. Some of the women talk like that—some of the single women say, 'I just don't know what to say when I say there is no father.' Well, that's impossible." There is always a father, although with donor insemination it is often hard for single women to explain pregnancy to others in the absence of any direct involvement with a man.

"What to Say About Daddy" is the hottest seminar Single Women by Choice puts on. As the children get older and more verbal, says founder psychotherapist Jane Mattes, herself the unmarried mother of a seven-year-old boy, they want to know about the man who isn't there. At least DI married women have a male "social" father, but in the case of single DI mothers, father is not there at all and never was.

Society will have to decide the answer to columnist Ellen Goodman's question: "What does it mean to deliberately bring a generation of fatherless children into the world?"

Unusual Families

Whereas single women, hetero- or homosexual, can avail themselves of the medically simple and inexpensive solution of artificial insemination, a man without a woman in his life has a more difficult time begetting a child he can call entirely his own.

Today, although many surrogate agencies restrict their services to married infertile couples, some do offer single men the chance of a surrogate baby.

Says Beth Bacon of the Hagar Institute, "When we were first contacted by a single man, we were really kind of floored. We had always thought about our services as being for infertile couples, but the more we thought about it, the more we decided it would be all right. Adoption agencies are nowadays placing children with single men and women, so we figured it would be all right. We also knew plenty of single men who were raising children alone as the result of divorce or the death of a spouse, and they seemed to be doing a fine job, so there was no reason to discriminate against single men."

The Hagar Institute would not *a priori* reject homosexual men. Noel Keane has provided surrogate babies to several single men, but he draws the line at homosexuals. However, he tried to arrange a surrogate birth for a woman who was born a male.

While some people may not object strenuously to letting a single heterosexual woman who failed to find a husband have children, many people would probably want to deprive homosexual men and women of the opportunity to bear and rear offspring. But, says Dr. Susan Robinson, talking about homosexual women, "The idea that alternative insemination should be restricted to married couples struck me as narrow-minded and unfair." She feels that any single woman's desires to have a family are as valid as those of married women.[14]

Providing insemination services for a lesbian violates basic societal taboos, tacking the sin of homosexuality on top of the original sin of a single woman, aiding and abetting the creation of a child by a person who doesn't practice normal sexual habits and normally wouldn't create one anyway.

"Homosexuality was essentially a sexual evil," notes Robert Whitehurst, editor, with Lester Kirkendall of *The New Sexual Revolution*, "because it did not have as its goal reproduction, the essence of the sex act to Christians. The detachment of love from marriage, the refusal of Roman women to bear children, high abortion rates, and a host of other nonsexual problems appear to have conspired in the downfall of Rome. . . . Rome fell, and our ancestry was in some measure determined by these established trends."[15]

"We have a mythical norm of what the appropriate family is," says sociologist Rona Achilles. "There are very few around, but it still stands as a very persistent norm. I know lots of single parents who do quite well. Their families may be emotionally more stable than some families where there is a father."

Many studies, according to Carson Strong of the University of Tennessee, indicate "that the homosexual aspect of the home environment does not have a negative effect on the child's behavior or future sexuality. Green, for example, investigated the question of whether children raised by lesbians had an increased tendency to become homosexual themselves. Among twenty-one children, it was found that twenty exhibited behavior typical of their sex. The children who reported erotic fantasies or overt sexual behavior were all heterosexually oriented."[16]

It may well be that genuine love of the child is ultimately more important for its well-being than the sexual orientation of its parents. But the further we move away from the traditional biological family, the more uneasy we get. When it comes to homosexuals and transsexuals, we are suddenly less concerned with the method of conception and more worried about the child's upbringing in an unorthodox environment. Surrogacy and DI open the possibility of letting almost anybody who can afford it have children. If it is no longer so much a question of infertility as who should be allowed to have a baby, where do we draw the line? When we think of homosexuals and transsexuals having children, we confront our deepest beliefs and prejudices, and we want to draw protective barriers around them—perhaps with good reason.

Children as Commodities

As soon as the normal biological barriers have been broken, children become a question not just of nature, but of economics. Are we turning children into commodities? We seem to be headed in that direction, and few of us like the thought. Most of us would agree with Larry Palmer, professor of family law at Cornell University Law School, who says, "I think having children . . . falls outside the scope of a market decision. Having a child is not the same as buying a used car."[17] Professor Palmer's remark is, of course, meant to shock a bit. Is there any validity to the comparison?

The question of children as a commodity comes up particularly strongly in the debate about surrogacy. Are surrogates selling and childless couples buying babies? Are they traders in human beings? Are they more mercenary and immoral than people who pay doctors thousands of dollars to make possible the conception of "high tech" babies? Those opposed to surrogacy think so and use the baby-selling argument to back up their demands for banning the practice, for clearly it is neither moral nor legal to sell children. Those who tolerate surrogacy because they understand the pain of childlessness say that surrogates are selling services, not babies.

Let's for a moment play a game of baby selling. Only answers based on logic are allowed in the first part of the game. All you have to do is answer yes or no.

Imagine a woman who wants a child. She has functioning ovaries but no uterus. Her husband has no fertility problems. A couple of years ago there was no way that they could have a baby of their own, but today they can take advantage of the advances in medical science and surrogacy and have an *in vitro* baby by a surrogate mother.

The infertile woman and her husband can go to a doctor who will extract one or more of the wife's eggs and fertilize them with the husband's sperm in a petri dish. But since the wife had no uterus, the embryo cannot be implanted in her body. However, the couple have signed up with a surrogate agency that has linked them up with a surrogate mother. For $10,000 the surrogate has agreed to have the embryo inserted into her womb via a catheter and to carry the fetus for nine months. (Several major hospitals in the United States offer that procedure, via what is sometimes called a "host uterus program." A handful of babies have been born by that method, and more are on the way.) The surrogate in this case does not supply an egg, she only provides a womb.

Is the surrogate selling the baby? A yes answer shows that your logic is faulty, because she cannot sell what is not hers in the first place—the egg isn't hers and neither is the sperm.

Is she selling her parental rights to the baby? Again, the correct answer is no. She is not the biological parent of the child, and she has not adopted the baby, so she has no parental rights to sell. She is renting a womb to the infertile couple and selling nutrition to the growing baby. In other words, her fee must be for rent of her womb and compensation for her time and discomfort.

Human life is created when a woman's egg fuses with a man's sperm. Are both an egg and a sperm equally essential to the creation of a baby? If your answer is no, get your parents to explain about the birds and the bees. If your answer is yes, proceed.

If a couple wants to have a child and the man is infertile, one solution to their infertility problem is for the woman to be inseminated with sperm of another man. The sperm can be fresh or it can be frozen and can be bought from one of the many sperm banks in this country. The man who donates his sperm receives approximately $50 for his ejaculate. Is the sperm donor selling his baby? Both a yes and a no answer allow you to go to the next question.

Suppose again that a couple wants to have a child but while the man is fertile the woman has a problem getting pregnant. She cannot produce an egg—because she was born without ovaries or had them removed as a result of disease or because her ovaries simply will not produce a normal egg. Modern medical science can help her. The physician can remove a ripe egg from another woman and fertilize that egg with the sperm of the infertile woman's husband in a petri dish. Once the egg has become an embryo, it can be implanted into the uterus of the infertile woman, who will carry the baby to term. (About forty babies have been born by this method and by the related technique of embryo transfer, which has resulted in about a dozen births.) If everything goes well, the embryo will attach itself to her uterine wall and grow into a normal baby, and nine months later she will give birth to a child. The child will carry the genes of the husband and the egg donor. The mother who actually gives birth is not related by blood to the child. The woman who donates the egg may receive about $250 as compensation for the egg and the physical pain and danger she submits herself to.

Are female egg donors (or embryo donors) selling their babies? If your answer is identical to your previous response, you get an extra point for logical consistency. If you answered no, you do not have a logical leg to stand on. The egg donor sells her baby to the same extent that a sperm donor sells his. Hobble back to start.

Readers who have kept their cool and suppressed all the buts, howevers, and neverthelesses, may now prepare themselves for the 10-point bonus question.

A "traditional" surrogate mother—although the tradition is only about a decade old—stands in for an infertile woman in all aspects of conception and pregnancy. She is inseminated with sperm of the infertile woman's husband; she provides the egg and carries the baby in her body for nine months, gives birth to it, and turns it over to the couple, who have paid her around $10,000 for her services.

Is *she* selling the baby? If you answer yes, you are still in the game, provided you answered yes to all the other questions of baby selling, but if you previously said no, you go back three questions. A traditional surrogate sells an egg just like female egg donors, and just like a sperm donor sells his sperm. A traditional surrogate rents out her womb, but so do *in vitro* surrogates. A traditional surrogate simply performs two services instead of one. If considered individually donating an egg and renting a womb do not amount to baby selling, then adding up the no's leaves you with no still.

If you feel that egg and sperm donors are selling babies, and that traditional surrogates are doing that, too, you are being logical and are entitled to your view.

Readers who have maintained their logical balance up to this point may now shake their fists and shout, "But . . . !"

Attitudes to surrogacy involve more than logic; emotional considerations may play a far greater role in our reactions to the practice. We feel uneasy about making babies in untraditional ways, and paying strangers for their help in a process that is extremely private somehow seems to cheapen a sacrosanct area of our lives.

Says Hilary Hanafin, a psychologist who screens surrogates in Los Angeles, "There is something very distressing about surrogates getting money, and it has hit a raw nerve. It has to do with the whole idea of women's bodies and babies. Any kind of money attached to that demoralizes it and dehumanizes it. I do think that people have an association that if you put money into something, it becomes less humanitarian."

That may be part of it, and yet we do not get upset at paying doctors thousands of dollars for *in vitro* fertilization, for instance, and do not give much thought to the reality that a sperm donor gets paid for masturbating into a jar. There is something else that bothers us with surrogacy, but we cannot quite put our finger on the emotional sore spot so resort to dramatic accusations of baby selling. Many who can logically lay the baby-selling argument to rest may still feel uncomfortable and object to surrogacy, but at least now they know they have to look for the answer to their uneasiness in their emotional makeup.

Surrogacy Compared to Private Adoption

Giving away babies is nothing new. Adoption is a practice that has probably gone on since the beginning of mankind. Adoption has been around for so long that it is a well-regulated and socially acceptable procedure. It has given innumerable unwanted or orphaned children a good life and has made thousands of childless couples happy. Few people, if any, have moral objections to it.

Adoptions in the United States used to be possible only through specific adoption agencies, and no money was allowed to change hands when a child was placed in a home. But adoption, like medical ways of having babies, has changed dramatically.

This ad, along with two others, appeared in the *Ithaca Journal* under the classified heading Adoptions.

A baby to adopt is our dream. Loving couple wants to give newborn love & a special life. Let us help you. All expenses paid. Legal and confidential. Please call Joe & Ellen, collect.

Joe and Ellen Learner, thirty-four and thirty-three, have been married for thirteen years. He is a facilities coordinator for IBM, and she is a contract administrator for West Point Military Academy. They live in a house the two of them "get lost in" in a small town about fifty miles from New York City. For seven years they have tried to have a child, but for undetermined reasons they have not succeeded. Joe checked out fine, and although the doctors could find nothing wrong with Ellen, she went through exploratory laparoscopies, an operation, and artificial insemination—all to no avail. They decided to adopt and went to several agencies, but there were no suitable babies available.

"They all give you the same line," says Ellen, "a five-year wait for a white infant. Get on the list."

The Learners did not want to wait that long and sought out a lawyer specializing in adoptions. He offered them more hope.

"There are a million teenagers having babies in this country every year," he told them. "All this business about a three- to five-year wait is baloney. Just get out there and find them."

Joe and Ellen have had a couple of responses to their ad, but nothing has worked out yet. It is a trying time; every time the phone rings they think, "This is going to be it."

Joe and Ellen are hoping to find a white infant who is not handicapped. They prefer a newborn but will accept a child who is up to two years old. They are looking for a young woman who is pregnant but does not want to keep the child. They will pay for her medical expenses through pregnancy and delivery, but nothing else. Their lawyer warned them: "Don't agree to give her any other money during the pregnancy. If she calls in the middle of the night and says, 'Pay me a hundred dollars or the deal is off,' say no. She will try to hold it over your head.' "

Joe and Ellen are attempting to get a child through private adoption, which is legal in thirty-five states. Such adoptions are nearly always expensive and sometimes risky. Mr. William Pierce, president of the National Committee on Adoption, estimates that at least a tenth of independent adoptions involve some illegal or unethical practice.[18]

Marketplace factors can enter into private adoption more easily than into surrogacy. Whereas a couple who contracts with a surrogate has worked out the question of payment before the baby is even conceived, a young woman who is already pregnant can promise the baby will go to the couple who gives her the best deal. Legally she can only have her medical expenses covered and be reimbursed for lost wages, but a lot can be slipped to her under the guise of gifts. The prospective parents can be outbid.

Of course, just as the biological mother can pick out the best customer, the couple can shop around for the kind of baby they want. A couple expecting a surrogate baby pays the biological mother whether or not the child is normal and even if it is stillborn, and they have to accept the baby. Adoptive parents can avoid being saddled with an unhealthy child. For a surrogate baby there is only one customer, whereas there are hundreds of eager adoptive parents vying for an infant already in the making. Marketplace pressures enter into adoption to a greater extent than in surrogacy, and it is easier to influence a young woman in a tough situation.

Says lawyer Matthew L. Myers when comparing adoption and surrogacy, "Don't kid yourself, because in many respects it is a question of semantics. [In private adoption] you find a woman with an unwanted pregnancy who is facing the stresses with very little support around her one way or the other, who suddenly finds herself blown back and forth with somebody throwing money at her to do something she may be uncomfortable with. [In surrogacy] the woman isn't pregnant when the process starts; she doesn't have any pressure other than the pressure she puts on herself before she becomes pregnant. She gets lots of opportunities to say, 'This is not something I want to do.' The abuse of private adoptions has the potential [for baby selling] to a much greater degree than surrogacy does—there is no question about that. The other side of it is, though, precisely because of the extraordinary fear that private adoption will turn into baby selling, virtually every state has laws carefully regulating it. Whether those laws are effective or enforced is another question.''

If Joe and Ellen find a pregnant girl who agrees to give up her child, they will sign a preliminary agreement with her specifying that she promises the child to them. They expect to meet the mother, to be in the hospital during the delivery, and to take the baby home as soon as it is discharged from the hospital. From then on, all contact will be cut off, very much like many surrogacy arrangements. However, the law in all states allows the biological mother a certain amount of time to change her mind—in New York State it is forty-five days—and waiting out those days can be very difficult for the adoptive parents.

The Learners will spend $300 to $400 dollars a month on ads, their lawyer gets a modest $3000, and while medical expenses for the biological mother cannot be estimated precisely, they hope to get a baby for a total of about $7,500.

"I've talked to these places in Georgia," Ellen says. "They wanted twenty-five thousand dollars—ten thousand dollars just to get them looking for you and fifteen thousand on the delivery of the baby. I have heard of a couple of places that high.''

The cost of a private adoption can easily be on a par with surrogacy, and the middleman gets all the money.

In many fundamental ways, private adoptions are very similar to surrogacy. An unborn child is promised away; the biological mother receives money; a lawyer, as with a surrogate agency, is paid to deal with formal matters; and the adoptive parents take the baby home immediately after birth.

We take private adoptions in stride in spite of the fact that the procedure may be much closer to baby selling than surrogacy is. The biological mother receives money for carrying and giving up a child already in the making—to put it crudely, there is a product to sell.

There are, however, two important factors that distinguish private adoptions from surrogacy: the child is entirely unrelated to the future parents and it was "not planned"—a nicer way of saying unwanted. Normally, many people would find the child's not being genetically related to its parents a slight drawback. And we feel a little sad that the baby is unwanted, although somehow it makes giving up the child seem less unnatural.

It is easy for us to imagine a young girl falling in love and getting caught in an unfortunate circumstance. Even the most moralistic of us can probably sympathize with the girl's situation, and we might even admire her for not taking the easy way out: abortion. We imagine the poor girl agonizing over what to do while she weighs the best interests of the child against her own maternal feelings. We are convinced that if there were any possible way, she would choose to bring up her child, but she is good-hearted and realizes that the child will have a better chance in a fine home all ready to receive and love the baby. We tell ourselves that she is being heroic and altruistic when she tears the child from her bosom, for it is her deep love of the child that enables her to give it up. She is doing the right thing, what is best for the baby. Never once do we allow ourselves to think that she might be indifferent to the baby and is giving it up without any emotional suffering.

Surrogacy deprives us of such fantasies; there are no mitigating circumstances. The surrogate knows even before the child is conceived that it will be given up—the child is planned and created for somebody else. Relinquishing the baby is a matter of premeditated surrender. It makes us queasy that a surrogate can take such a calculated approach to a baby that is partly her own flesh and blood because we do not like to acknowledge the possibility that there may not be a deep unbreakable bond between mother and child.

Says psychologist Hilary Hanafin, "I think surrogate moms are challenging some of our ideas about what women are and what women can do. They feel that women have been stereotyped. Not every woman feels exactly the same way about every child she carries; the degree of attachment that occurs between a woman and a fetus varies quite a bit. It is a twentieth-century male notion that every woman feels absolutely and invariably an attachment to every fetus she carries. If that were the case, we would not have abortion. Surrogates basically say, 'I can feel different about this pregnancy than I do about the other.' Women should not be commanded to feel absolute attachment."

Even old-fashioned mothers who want to have and keep their own baby may not feel an immediate surge of love for their newborn child. According to Marshall Klaus, a California expert on maternal infant bonding, "Roughly twenty-five percent of normal mothers begin to feel the baby is theirs when they are carrying it, and twenty-five percent feel it is theirs within an hour of birth, and then another forty percent take a week or more." Furthermore, he says, "it could be useful exploring the idea that you don't become hooked immediately. It is not epoxy bonding."

Sometimes bonding is instantaneous; sometimes it can take a lot longer to occur. However, a note of caution from Klaus: "The more one explores what it is like for a mother to give up a baby, the more one is impressed that it is not an easy question." In fact, there are no easy answers, but because society assumes an instant and deep attachment, mothers tend to keep a slow maternal response a secret.

The idea of absolute mother-child attachment may well be a relatively modern notion originating among middle class women in the late eighteenth century, when "the romantic cult of motherhood fixed these women in their homes, assigning them the care and upbringing of their infants, while their husbands concerned themselves with money and career."[19] Before that new concept of motherhood got entrenched, mothers found it quite acceptable to send their newborn babies to a wet nurse in the country immediately after birth. Wet-nursing has been a Western custom since antiquity, and the practice survived in many regions into early modern times. In France it was a commercialized cottage industry until after World War I. However, already in the mid-eighteenth century, moralists such as the philosopher Jean-Jacques Rousseau campaigned against wet-nursing, calling it a crime against nature and a sign of social corruption. Like most twentieth-century Americans, he saw mothering as the natural function of a woman.

Wet-nursing eventually went the way of blood-letting, but for an upper class European child the nanny took over where the wet nurse left off. Children saw their parents for a few minutes a day, during which they were expected to be on their best behavior. Parents generally subscribed to the rule that children should be seen and not heard. Parents were remote and sometimes feared figures. Winston Churchill, for instance, had a distant admiration for his mother and the deepest attachment to his beloved nanny all through his life.

Having been brought up in the romantic tradition of motherhood, we may in retrospect feel that wet-nursing and turning over the upbringing of a child to its nanny are unnatural, but even today we do not behave all that differently. A large number of modern American families consist of children and two wage earners, both of whom are away from the home most of the child's waking hours. This is true in many cases even while the child is an infant. Not infrequently, the mother goes back to work soon after the birth and leaves her infant in full-time day care. We entrust most of the care of our newborn children to others. We may not prefer it that way, but we do it and accept it.

If we are willing to tolerate the daily separation of parents from small children, who often cry for their absent mommies, why do we find it so unnatural that a mother would be prepared in advance to give up her baby, to separate from a newborn child she has not even gotten to know? It seems that a modern woman is expected to feel as much attachment for a child still in her womb as to one already born. We balk at the idea of a surrogate mother "baby-sitting" an unborn child but find it quite acceptable to pay a woman to care for our own clinging, crying infants. Many mothers who would probably prefer to bring up their own children do not, and yet society does not consider them morally suspect. Probably all couples who have surrogate babies would prefer to have their own. The difficulty is that they cannot.

Notes Rhonda Billig, legal counsel for Resolve, "Surrogacy is nobody's first choice. Most have gone through years of tests. The popular misconception is that people do this as a selfish choice."[20]

When people with no other choice have surrogate babies, society is apt to be morally upset even though the unborn child does not mind and the future parents are happy about the arrangement.

If the people involved in surrogacy—the surrogate mother, the future parents, the agencies, and probably the baby, who would not have had a life any other way—find this method of having children acceptable, why are the rest of us, who are just bystanders, objecting to it?

"One thing to remember," says Hanafin, "is that a surrogate giving away a child hits at the core of our universal and individual beliefs about mothers and attachment. If we take a larger psychological perspective, the fact that surrogates give away babies really says to us on some very deep unconscious level that maybe moms and babies aren't eternally attached one hundred percent. That is a direct threat to my attachment with my mother and your attachment with your mother and everybody's attachment with their mother. As small children we really need to believe that Mommy's love is invariable and absolute, and surrogates are saying what we don't want to hear—that Mommy's love is conditioned on who Daddy was, how she got pregnant, how she felt about you—that she could give you away if the time and place were right. We hate to confront the notion that mother-and-child attachment is not an absolute, because that is a personal threat to all of us.''

Surrogacy and the Law

Even if surrogacy is no more baby-selling than private adoption, we still do not like it that money is involved in the transaction. "Surrogacy is appalling to a lot of people," says Resolve's Billig, who nevertheless thinks "it is important to maintain surrogacy as an option. It's nice to think it's altruistic . . . but we feel the financial remuneration is important. If you take away the money, we don't feel the donors will be there. You might as well prohibit the practice altogether, if you are going to prohibit the money."[21]

The Push for Prohibition

Prohibiting the money is one strategy that many people see as useful in discouraging surrogacy, and that is precisely the policy that has been adopted in England. Said Dame Mary Warnock, head of the Warnock Commission, which issued its report in July 1984, "There are now waiting in America a largish number of agencies wishing and anxious to start on this side of the Atlantic, and I think there is a market for such agencies. I regard it as a matter of extreme urgency that to set up such agencies should be made a criminal offense . . . people are not prepared to have in this country agencies which exploit both the misery of the infertile and the willingness of women to act as surrogates."[22]

When the Surrogacy Arrangements Bill was debated in the House of Commons, the Minister for Health, Mr. Kenneth Clarke, reported that "a contract would be regarded as unenforceable by the courts and contrary to public policy."[23]

The Surrogacy Arrangements Act of 1985 outlawed all commercial arrangements and agencies, as well as advertising designed to bring together surrogates and commissioning couples.[24]

In the United States, the state of Louisiana has adopted similar laws, but there is little chance that surrogacy, already so well established in this country, will be discouraged out of existence by such laws. What is more likely to happen is that new Baby M cases will be dragged through custody court, for as Dame Warnock observed, "The courts do, however, have jurisdiction over children which is quite separate from and independent of the law of contract. Where a court has to consider the future of a child born following a surrogacy agreement, it must do so in accordance with the child's best interests in all the circumstances of the case, and not according to the terms of any agreement between various adults. The child's interests being the first and paramount consideration, it seems likely that only in very few exceptional circumstances would a court direct a surrogate mother to hand over the child to the commissioning couple. The present state of the law makes any surrogacy agreement a risky undertaking for those involved."[25]

"I admire the position that the Warnock Commission took," says ethicist John Fletcher. "Morally, I think, it is the right position. Surrogacy is a great act of kindness and ought to be modestly encouraged, particularly for medical reasons, but I think the commercial aspect of surrogacy ought to be discouraged. Surrogacy could be kept within the limits of the framework of management of medical problems and defined more appropriately as a way to overcome a genetic disease or extreme cases of infertility. I see these spin-offs into commercial solutions as very unfortunate."

Several people have suggested that surrogacy laws should be similar to those regulating organ donation.

Says Professor Larry Palmer, "My general view of surrogacy is that it is something that should be allowed but not necessarily encouraged. Like organ transplants, it is something we allow but don't encourage. We don't allow people to sell their organs. It is morally offensive. There are certain things society chooses to distribute in ways other than the marketplace. There are some things we want people to give away, and organs are that because they relate to a social construct, health. It violates our ideals as a society if we don't live as if everyone gets the same health care. We want everybody to have it, so we provide it for free."

It would make us feel better about surrogacy if everybody—rich and poor alike—who could not have a baby any other way would be provided one free of charge through the health system. If surrogacy agreements were to be "worked out through the assistance of medically competent people who are dealing with medical problems," as Fletcher suggests, it would certainly eliminate a lot of, in Fletcher's words, "the pirates operating off the coast of health care, who are making pious noises about their services," but then, in all likelihood, nobody would get a surrogate baby. A health system that cannot even supply the most basic medical care to poor people is not about to distribute babies in an equitable way. As long as medical services are ruled by market forces, it seems unreasonable that doctors should be paid for their part in producing surrogate babies, while the women who take the actual risks and do all the "work" are expected to provide their services for free. In a system allowing for little reward for surrogate mothers, few women would be available, and the shortage might well force the practice underground.

Surrogacy is already so entrenched in this country that efforts to ban the practice or greatly reduce it are probably going to be unsuccessful. It might be more realistic to pass laws that would set reasonable limits on how far it can go.

Whose Baby Is It?

Even if states were to follow the British example, legislation banning surrogacy would clearly be inadequate for dealing with new variations of the practice. In instances where the surrogate mother is carrying a child created from the "commissioning" couple's egg and sperm, it is not clear who the legal mother of the child is. The surrogate has no genetic stake in the baby, but she has given birth to it. Points out Judge Marianne O. Battani of Wayne County Circuit Court, "We really have no definition of 'mother' in our law books. Mother was supposed to have been so basic that no definition was deemed necessary."[26]

In the situation where a woman gives birth to a child that she is genetically completely unrelated to, as in *in vitro* surrogacy, the question of who the mother is is particularly complicated. Is the woman who provided the egg the mother, or is it the woman who carried the child and gave birth to it? Noel Keane, who has arranged a few *in vitro* surrogacy births, went to court before the birth of one baby to get an answer. The court agreed with Keane's request to declare the genetic parents the legal parents of the baby.

Other people do not agree with that decision. Professor Palmer and Professor George Annas prefer to work on the assumption that the woman who gives birth to the baby is the legal mother regardless of the genetic origin of the child, thus leaving it up to her to sign over the baby to another set of parents or not.

Says Palmer, "Once a child is born, it *prima facie* belongs to the woman who gave birth to it. It belongs to her until she gives it away, and there is no way you can force her to give it away, because she is in control of her own reproduction." Palmer feels that no matter what the genetic origin of the child, a contract cannot deprive the birth mother of the right to keep the child if she so chooses. "There are some things we do not allow people to contract about. We do not allow people to contract about babies. We have a concept of children that is an obligation beyond contract. You are a parent, you are intrinsically bound with that other person in a covenant. Feelings about children are irrational. If we look at Mary Beth Whitehead from the perspective of a contract, she looks like a stupid, dizzy female. If you look at her as someone who cares for a child's life [then her behavior is understandable]. It has to be an almost irrational attachment. You don't want to kill that; A contract is a rational process, a covenant changes your being."

Palmer would like to see the situation structured so that the law "allows this giveaway to happen—and you can pay, but the money would be for her time and medical expenses." He would also like to see a law that in cases of surrogacy "shortens the time for adoption, three days, and once she gives it up, that's it."

Lori Andrews wants not even three days of legal limbo after the child is born. "I think with respect to surrogacy, the time in which the decision should be final should be before or at the birth of the child," she says. "There should not be time for the surrogate to change her mind. I think a different policy [than for adoption] is justified because of the different circumstances. A woman who is pregnant is in a different situation than a woman who is deciding whether or not to become a surrogate. A potential surrogate can take as long as she wants to make that decision; she isn't faced with the *fait accompli* of an existing pregnancy about which she has to make a difficult choice. It would be an added safeguard to have judicial scrutiny in advance, but whether you do it through that mechanism or through other assurances of informed consent, I would uphold the contract."

There is no doubt that the commissioning couple and agencies would like to see legislation to that effect, and many surrogates would, too.

Keane surrogate Donna Regan favors prejudicial consent.

"It means," she explains, "that you go before a judge after the medical and psychiatric testing, and he asks if you are giving informed consent. You can either say yes or no, and he determines whether you are or aren't. I think that's all that's necessary. From that point it is a legally binding contract."

But, argues Michigan lawyer Wiley Bean, regardless of what the contract says, the relation between surrogate and couple is always going to be unequal in terms. "The sperm donor doesn't have to take the child if he doesn't want to," he says. "All he has to say is that if it is my child, I will be responsible for child support. The sperm donor doesn't have to take the child, you can't force him to take the child. You can get specific performance from only one side. The obligation to support can be enforced, the obligation to parent cannot."

Beth Bacon of the Hagar Institute has never come across a case where the biological father refused the child. "I would sooner worry that the seas would cover the earth," she says, but, of course, that does not mean it could not happen. "Our people have been through a very thorough screening process, and we talk with each couple about all the horrible what-ifs— What if you got a divorce, who would get the child? What if the husband dies in a car wreck while the surrogate is pregnant, would you still want the baby? What if they both did? It is in the contract that they have to put who they want to raise the baby—they have to make that decision ahead of time. If we ever did have that circumstance, we are a licensed child placement agency, and we certainly know hundreds of couples who would be wonderful parents and desperate for a child, and that baby would be placed in a wonderful home. Of course, the surrogate might decide to keep the child. But this is the last thing I lose sleep over."

Even if the biological father cannot be forced to bring up his child, he can at least be forced to support it, so as abhorrent as it may seem to take a contract out on a child—it sounds like a Mafia modus operandi—it may be in the best interests of the baby. If society sincerely wants to put the welfare of the child above the wishes of the surrogate and the contracting couple, it will try to avoid litigation over who has a right to the child while it is being carted back and forth between the warring parties. The child is better off if there is no discussion of where it belongs; the parents are better off; and the surrogate is better off, because if she knows the contract is binding, she is less likely to get into an arrangement that she is not 100 percent sure she can handle.

The Rights of the Surrogate During Pregnancy

Badly needed definitions and legislation of any kind are slow in coming. While the question of who has the right to a surrogate child is central, the law also needs to deal with the rights and obligations between the couple and the surrogate during pregnancy.

Critics of surrogacy have argued that a surrogate signs away fundamental rights to the degree that in reality she enslaves herself for nine months.

It is illegal for any human being to give him- or herself in slavery in the United States, regardless of whether the person freely chooses to do so. The slavery argument is "specious," as attorney Matthew Meyers puts it, but there are serious questions as to how much control the couple or an agency who contracts with a surrogate can exert over her life.

In her testimony before a congressional committee on May 21, 1987, Lori Andrews gave her view of the matter: "Some surrogate contracts claim to give the couple the right to force the surrogate to follow doctor's orders, to undergo amniocentesis and have an abortion (or not have an abortion) based on their desires. A law proposed in Michigan a few years ago would have prohibited a surrogate from smoking or drinking during pregnancy. Such contracts and laws overlook the fact that the surrogate has a right to bodily integrity. It is inappropriate for the government to set standards on women's behavior during pregnancy."

What if a contract has a statement that a woman must undergo amniocentesis and she refuses? "Is she liable for negligence?" asks Stacy DeBroff, author of the "National Staff Surrogate Paper" for the American Civil Liberties Union. "That puts the health of the fetus above the health of the mother. If the surrogate wants an abortion, can the father force her to carry it to term? We have a hard time sorting out individual liberties."[29]

Although many surrogate contracts do contain prohibitions against drinking and smoking and order the surrogate to eat right—and also demand that she have an abortion, should the couple want it—they are probably not and should probably not be enforceable either in practice or in a court of law. As unpleasant as it may be for the couple, the surrogate's fundamental rights have to be respected. The uncertainties that may arise as a result are part of the inherent dangers of surrogacy.

Many states have surrogacy legislation on the drawing board that would deal with the question of contracts, when the surrogate would have to make a decision, payment, etc., but also about who can enter into surrogate agreements.

Suggested legislation for the District of Columbia, introduced by councilman John Ray, would, among other things:

• Establish that a couple entering into an agreement with a surrogate mother will have all parental rights and responsibilities for the child, regardless of the condition of the child, and the surrogate mother will have no parental rights or responsibilities

• Set twenty-five as the minimum age for anyone entering into a surrogate parenting agreement
• Define standards for screening out potential sperm donors and participants in surrogate parenting agreements who have sexually transmitted diseases and genetic disorders
• Require surrogate parenting centers to be licensed
• Require informed consent
• Prohit surrogate parenting centers from advertising that the technologies will result in a child with superior physical or genetic traits[28]

Ray's bill will probably run into opposition from people who will want much tighter restrictions. His suggestion leaves the door open for untraditional parenting arrangements. Surrogacy is feared as a threat to the already besieged American family. The question is, should surrogacy be restricted to heterosexual infertile married couples? That may at first thought seem a reasonable requirement, but wouldn't such a law be more conservative than the society it regulates?

And yet, without legal limits, the future of surrogacy could take an unsavory turn.

Traditional surrogacy does not conjure up brave new world images because medically it is simple and quite natural, requiring only artificial insemination. Popular worries about women turning into breeding machines seem much exaggerated. A woman's child-bearing capacity is limited, so there are natural boundaries to how efficient a child-producing factory any one woman can become. However, the minute fertile women begin to think it is a good idea to have surrogate babies for convenience, we get into iffy territory.

Abortion may tell us what can happen. Abortion is unrestricted during the first trimester of pregnancy. Any woman can have an abortion for any reason whatsoever. Dr. Mark Geier encountered a case where a woman terminated a pregnancy because it would interfere with her vacation plans, and there have probably been abortions for even more frivolous reasons, although it is hard to think of one. If no restrictions are placed on surrogacy, it is entirely possible that perfectly healthy, fertile women may find it more convenient to have somebody else produce a child for them. A model might lose income while pregnant and get her body permanently marred by stretch marks; a busy executive would be encumbered by a big stomach and project the wrong image. So why not pay somebody to do it? The objections to using a surrogate for such and similar reasons are as strong as objections to abortion for convenience.

It is cause for concern, but surrogacy combined with new medical techniques offers truly unpleasant possibilities.

The Question of Genetic Engineering

The spectre of eugenics raises its pretty and intelligent head. For several years it has been possible to flush out the embryo of a prize cow, one that gives an extraordinary amount of milk, for instance, and implant it into the womb of an ordinary, proletarian cow. In that way the prize cow can be the mother of thousands of superior calves in her lifetime. That technique, embryo transfer, can and has been used in humans so far only to overcome infertility, but it is entirely possible for a beautiful and smart woman to donate several eggs every menstrual cycle, and once the egg freezing techniques have been perfected, her eggs could be out in cold storage and offered for sale to anybody who wants to buy them.

Already, a couple who wants a good-looking little genius can go to the Repository for Germinal Choice, a sperm bank that collects ejaculate from Nobel prize winners and other superiorly endowed men. The physician can put a superior egg with the superior sperm in a petri dish and implant the resulting embryo into any other agreeable woman who is a good nurturer. Voila! The human race is improved without any discomfort to the genetic parents of the child. One egg donor and one sperm donor may produce exemplary offspring and be a popular choice—everybody will want one of the wonder babies—and donors have the capacity to produce hundreds of babies spread around the country. Just as people have title searches done before buying a house, a young couple in the future may have to do a parental search to make sure that they are not, in fact, biological brothers and sisters. Without strict legal limits, such a scenario is not so farfetched. One can imagine the day when a reproduction center will send out mail order catalogs describing the genetic characteristics of eggs and sperm in their freezer, and of the carrier women on call. The financially able customer can then make his or her choices, and receive a baby in the mail nine months later, courtesy of the United States Postal Stork Service.

The more we fiddle with reproduction outside the framework of a couple, the more we allow entreprenuers to get into the act of creation, the more we risk removing children from the concept of love and responsibility. We are likely to turn human beings into commodities and devalue life.

Such scenarios are easily avoidable with proper legislation and are not in and of themselves a reason to ban surrogacy. We may not want to allow all "capitalistic acts between consenting adults," in the words of the philosopher Robert Nozick, but surrogacy as such does not seem to undermine our ethical underpinnings.

Says John Fletcher, "Morally I see no fundamental reason to object to surrogacy. Once you're over the magic line of contraception, you're skiing down the slope. I don't see this as a slope down; in fact, I see it as a slope up. The burden of proof is on the people who want to stop it and to prove that it causes more misery than benefits."

The Objections to High-Tech Babies

Surrogacy is such an emotional issue for many people that reason goes on the blink and the debate occasionally gets overheated and ugly. The general public may feel equally uneasy about *in vitro* fertilization and related techniques, but perhaps because it is all oh-so-scientific, a lot of us feel left out of the discussion. We do not even speak the language. Eggs and sperm are gametes that form embryos in petri dishes in the process of extracorporeal fecundication. When scientists looking at the future talk about DNA, genomes, chromosomes, and restriction enzymes, the ordinary mind gets lost in double helixes and the jargon of the initiated. We do not completely understand the language, and the processes remain obscure as well, so even if we have strong negative intuitions, we are not about to make fools of ourselves by babbling about worries over something only dimly grasped. Most of us hope for the best and leave it to the scientists.

But the consequences of high-tech fertilization may be far more portentous than the ramifications of surrogacy, and they come upon us at break-neck speed. Says Dr. Gary Hodgen, "The interim time between discovery and application is so fast that the public doesn't have time to dialogue to it. . . . Society doesn't have a chance to examine or learn about anything because we put it on the railroad tracks with a rocket tied to it and it goes zoom, straight to the market because there are big bucks in it."

Already in 1984, the British magazine the *Economist* worried about the potential of the new birth technologies: "Human beings will end the second millennium since Christ perfecting new means to tamper, for the first time, with their own nature and existence. Having first unlocked the power to annihilate every living person already born, scientists are now learning new ways to meddle with the unborn. . . . Science is knowledge. Knowledge cannot be unlearnt. That is the present nuclear misfortune and it is the present genetic risk.''[29]

Church Opposition

Even though there is little popular debate about the scientific approach to babies, there are groups who out of philosophical rather than medical concerns wish to ban new ways of making babies. Foremost among these groups is the Catholic Church. In a surprising alliance of strange bedfellows, some feminists—for their own and different reasons—have joined forces with that paternalistic institution.

For years the Vatican has opposed birth control, which prevents a baby from being born. But creating a baby by external fertilization where none was possible before seems a life-affirming act, so why is the church against it?

The Catholic Church, Charles Krauthammer says, "opposes everything: *in vitro* fertilization, embryo freezing, embryo transfer, surrogate motherhood, artificial insemination not just by donor but by husband. The church sees what hell lies at the bottom of the slippery slope, and rather than erect bulwarks, detours, and sandbags, it declares the whole mountain off-limits.''[30] In the church's view, the slippery slope begins with the severing of "the inseparable connection . . . between the two meanings of the conjugal act: the unitive meaning and the procreative meaning,'' and thus rules out everything from birth control to *in vitro* fertilization.

Ethicist John Fletcher does not agree: "The biological unity is supposed to be representative of the spiritual unity between the couple. The error in this reasoning is that it elevates biology to a level of preeminence in theology that it should never have. It makes a kind of biological theology. The fault in this is idolatry, because it elevates something biological to a supernatural realm.''

To people who have practiced birth control for years, separating the unitive and procreative meaning of lovemaking is only a worry if they fail at it, and for infertile couples who desperately want a child, the conjugal act has already, to their dismay, lost it procreative meaning. The Vatican's prohibitions do not seem to loom large in the conscience of most people. But even so, the 'miracle of life' does seem to lose some of its meaning when lovemaking is replaced by a medical procedure, when people become reduced to laboratory animals, and egg and sperm become just raw materials that scientists mix in petri dishes according to a recipe.

Dr. Robert Stillman at George Washington University concedes that advances in medical ways of creating life "are taking some of the wonder and fascination out of it. But obviously from a scientific point of view, while the unknown and wonder are fascinating, they have their limitations, because what it means is that you don't understand."

A lack of understanding, of course, means a lack of control over the process.

"People separate nature into two categories—those things outside of our control and those things under our control," writes Jeremy Rifkin, a well-known opponent of the new birth technologies. "Those things we can't control we tend to regard as sacred. . . . As parts of nature come under our control, we desacralize them, turning them into mere utilities. In other words, the part of the becoming process that cannot be anticipated and manipulated remains in the realm of the sacred; the part that can be anticipated and made to serve human ends becomes profane. . . . It is also true that familiarity breeds contempt or indifference. As we gain control over things, they lose their fascination for us. What once was the object of our fear and respect becomes a mundane appendage. . . ."[31]

Normally children are conceived in a moment of passionate love, but emotions are banned from *in vitro* conceptions, and necessary detachment takes their place.

Says Betty Petersen, who had *in vitro* twins, "In order to cope with it emotionally, you have to start looking at it as a process. There is no emotion involved when you look at it as a step-by-step procedure. You have to look at it as simple office calls rather than creating a baby."

"*Desacralization* is a code word for deadening," writes Rifkin. "We adamantly maintain ourselves as subject and reduce everything else to object. . . . Detachment and desacralization go together."[32]

Any infertile couple resorting to noncoital conception would heatedly argue that while the process of creating life in a lab may be "desacralizing" and "deadening," it requires more love and determination than ordinary conception.

"What do you call what we went through!" Betty exclaims. "There was a lot of love in that. It has strengthened our marriage and brought us closer to God."

Feminists and the Issue of Control

God does not play a large role in the opposition of some feminists to the new birth technologies. They are worried about surrendering control of their lives to the medical establishment, and control is what feminism is all about. But strangely enough, it is the same fear of losing control that impels infertile women to seek out medical help.

"I hated myself—my body for failing me," said one woman. "It angered me that I could not control the 'house I live in'—my body."[33]

Another infertile woman who went through *in vitro* in an attempt to get pregnant began to ask herself, "Am I just doing this to gain control over the situation or do I really want a baby? I did begin to question whether I was really just so obsessed with it because I wanted to get pregnant and have a baby or because I wanted to get pregnant and have control over my body. It took me a long time trying to relate to being a mother."

So these women go to the doctor and try everything he—or in rare cases, she—has to offer in order to get back in control of their own fate. But the minute they begin treatment, they enter a twilight zone where their bodies are taken over by doctors, medication, charts, and machinery. To get their bodies to conform to their wishes, they surrender almost completely to science. The patient's only power lies in saying no, but saying no ends her chance of being mistress of her own house, her body. It is a bizarre situation.

Feminists like Gena Corea see a danger in relinquishing so much power to the medical establishment. She believes that the "language of therapy used in describing IVF obscures the fact that medicine is not just a healing art but is also an institution of social control. IVF gives the power structure potent tools for such control . . . that will reduce women to breeders and offer a centralized group of white men control over who is born into the world. This would not necessarily be a conspiracy or even a conscious policy. The efforts of diverse men to create technologies that will increase male control over women and reproduction may be unformalized and intuitive, but nonetheless effective."[34]

Although Corea probably overstates her case and certainly overlooks the fact that some of the pioneers of IVF in Britain, Australia, and America were women, in the long perspective there may be reason to look at birth technologies with a jaundiced feminine eye.

Bearing children is a woman's fundamental and most awe-inspiring power. It makes her a natural force and part of the rhythm of things. For thousands of years people have worshipped fertility goddesses in the image of the human mother. Like the planet, itself known as Mother Earth, which yielded crops when watered by the rain and dried by the wind, women, before the function of sperm was discovered, seemed to be impregnated by natural forces with little assistance from men. The fertile woman was a powerful creature.

There is little doubt that in most cultures in the world men have sought to control that power, primarily through the institution of marriage. The Christian church has done its best to regulate women's sexuality, to curtail this power by pretending that it sprang from other sources. Early Christians maintained that human beings were not really born until they had been baptized, and the church, a patriarchal institution if there ever was one, became "the mother of us all," as Paul declared in the New Testament.

"The priests of the society preside, or at least they did in the past," says John Fletcher. "The modern state got the religious leaders off the backs of people, first when it comes to deciding whom you should marry—your daddy could no longer pick your mate for you. Number two, getting a divorce; and number three, teaching people what is ethically right and wrong about sex. Whoever has the control of the ethics of sexuality has a very great deal of power in society."

The modern priests of science, perhaps encouraged by the worshippers of manna, have picked up where the church left off. Traditionally, birth attendants were midwives, women, but with the development of medical science, they were replaced by male physicians who campaigned to have childbirth taken out of the home and put in the hospital. Delivery was no longer a natural phenomenon but a medical event that doctors monitored and controlled. Women were doped up with painkillers and not even conscious at the birth of their children. Cesarean sections, which are heavily overused (partly due to threats of malpractice if a perfect baby is not delivered), further increased the physician's power and made women feel that childbirth was none of their business. Now, of course, control may start even before conception.

The eventual outcome of the new birth technologies may well be that women are no longer needed to gestate a baby. Physicians can already keep extremely premature babies alive, and every day they make advances in growing babies outside the mother's body. As scientists learn to take over the function of the womb and keep "unfinished" babies alive, and once teams of *in vitro* doctors become allowed and able to grow embryos in the laboratory for a longer time, the time needed for a fetus to inhabit the natural environment of the uterus will be narrowed. Eventually the neonatologist and the *in vitro* physician will join their skills and make natural gestation unnecessary. In the future, babies may be grown from beginning to end in an artificial womb, and the power structure, presumably dominated by men, will have robbed women of their fundamental power.

"If I were an embryologist, I should be eager for the day when I could actually see, let's say through a glass container, a conceptus develop from fertilization through to term," says Professor Joseph Fletcher. "It seems to me that what is known as artificial gestation . . . in such a nonuterine container is the most desirable thing in the world for me to imagine . . . Great thing . . . I hope it comes to pass soon. I think it will."[35]

The views and enthusiasm of Professor Fletcher do send a chill down the female spine, and feminist Robyn Rowland smells a rat. The position of women is being undermined.

"What may be happening," she says, "is the last battle in the long war of men against women. Women's position is most precarious . . . we may find ourselves without a product of any kind with which to bargain. For the history of 'mankind' women have been seen in terms of their value as childbearers. We have to ask, if that last power is taken away and controlled by men, what role is envisaged for women in the new world? Will women become obsolete? Will we be fighting to retain or reclaim the right to bear children—has patriarchy conned us once again? I urge you, sisters, to be vigilant."[36]

When artificial insemination became common, men had the same worries. As attorney Russell Scott wrote in 1981, "If reproduction by AI became the norm, it would follow that the human male would cease to be socially necessary. . . . The human species could easily be reproduced from stored sperm, or from sperm taken from a small number of selected living donors. The social implications of the disappearance of the historic role of the human male are difficult to imagine."[37]

For physiological reasons, men's reproductive power has always been more alienable than that of women. Men's involvement in the creation of a baby can stop after ejaculation, whereas up to now women's secret inner recesses have always been needed for the sperm to produce a result. But science has now robbed women of many of their reproductive secrets. The modern infertile woman may be to blame.

Dr. Stillman holds women's liberation partly responsible for the development and proliferation of new birth technologies.

"I think it has had a significant impact in two regards. It has made it much more necessary to have infertility services because of delay in childbirth. Also, I think women's attitudes towards health care both from a consumer point of view and the point of view of biological function of a woman, in this case reproduction, has made a greater demand on services that can help infertility, help conception. As women become more vocal and forceful in economics, political power structures, and in law and medicine as well, they are going to push to have these services available.''

The debate about birth technologies involves "a lot of issues about our vision of womanhood. That's what it is all about," says Wendy Chavkin, director of the office of Maternity Services in New York City. "Are some women pursuing all of this because they feel worthless if they can't produce a child? That's very disturbing to me.''

In one line of thinking, the irony of infertile women pursuing babies through high technology is, of course, that while they regain their basic value as childbearers, they also yield control to a largely male power structure.

Children are the one resource society, nations, and indeed the human race cannot do without, and as long as women are needed to provide them, they hold a bargaining chip they have never fully used in their struggle for liberation. But the ironies abound. A woman's inalienable power—at least for the time being—has also been the reason for her suppression. Not being able to control her fertility, she was trapped by childbearing and child rearing while men ran the world. Women's biological destiny has been their undoing.

Some feminists fear they will be victimized by the new birth technologies, but radical feminist Shulamith Firestone, taking an aggressive stance, welcomes high tech and uses it as a weapon. In the *Dialectics of Sex* she argues that the ultimate cause of inequality between the sexes is the different reproductive roles between men and women, and she sees liberation on the bottom of a petri dish and pins her hope on complete gestation outside the womb.

She writes, "I submit, then, that the first demand for any alternative system must be: (1) the freeing of woman from the tyranny of their reproductive biology by every means available, and the diffusion of the childbearing and child rearing role to the society as a whole, men as well as women."[38]

Demanding that men bear children may not be as farfetched as it sounds. Scientists have already succeeded in growing offspring within the abdominal cavity of male monkeys.

Obviously, women like Shulamith Firestone do not believe that their greatest value lies in the ability to bear children. They take it for granted that they have as much to offer in other areas of life as do men.

Few women would go as far as Firestone in their view of

scientific procreation, but there are sympathizers. Feminist Nancy Breeze is one, and she embraces the new technology in a very motherly way, saying, "Two thousand years of morning sickness and stretch marks have not resulted in liberation for women and children. If you should run into a petri dish, it could turn out to be your best friend. So rock it; don't knock it."[39]

Fate of Embryos

Innovative ways of creating babies allow us to control what we could not control before; reproductive science allows us to know what we did not know before. The result is choices that we could not have dreamed of a few years ago but that also increase our responsibilities.

"In the past we made choices without awareness or concern about hereditary and evolutionary consequences," says Clifford Grobstein. "Today certain choices are being presented for which we can no longer shift responsibility, whether to Divinity, Chance, or Unkind Fate."[40]

There has been something of a reversal in the old adage "Man proposes but God disposes. Now more than ever man disposes. Today we have many new ways of outwitting God and nature that may seem desirable to some people and dangerous to many others.

While physicians with a certain professional detachment perform egg snatches on women, while embryos divide in petri dishes in about 200 labs all over the country, while infertile couples keep their fingers crossed and legislatures lumber into slow action, we can all ponder whether, if a little knowledge is a dangerous thing, more knowledge may not be more dangerous.

In *Knowledge and the Future of Man,* John T. Edsall writes, "Some scientists and philosophers have said that science is ethically neutral, without influence on human values—that it is significant only as a tool, enabling us to realize our aims more effectively but in itself without influence on the nature of those aims. That I do not believe. . . . as science grows, as our picture of the world and of man is enlarged and deepened by it, and as its consequences for the world become ever more apparent, it becomes one of the major forces that modifies and remolds our concept of what is good, what is tolerable, and what is intolerable in human life and conduct. These are not abstract issues; they involve many of the deepest personal and social conflicts of our time."[41]

There is no denying that science and technology have a profound impact on the world, and although our modern lifestyles depend on the fruits of science, many of us nevertheless fear the implications of new technologies, taking it for granted that the impact is likely to be negative.

But, says John Fletcher, "You can bend over backwards and spend a lifetime condemning technology that would never have been used in the past, and you don't see that there is a fit sometimes between technological advances and help on the ethical level."

Medical schools, propelled by increasing questions raised by the fast-paced nature of technological innovations, have established bio-ethics programs that gather panels to ponder the implications of new birth technologies and address questions such as how embryos should be taken care of in the lab, what type of experimentation is justified, who should have access to new types of infertility treatments, and what the potential is for improving human life and for abuses. These questions, which have no obvious answers, are matters of ethics, and "when we speak of ethics, we're talking about the rules people are expected to obey in their future actions."[42]

In their rich hormonal solution embryos created outside the womb float between being and nothingness. When they have reached the eight-cell stage, some of them will be transferred back into the wombs of women who hope that they will attach themselves to their uterine wall and grow into normal babies. Some of them will not. Via hormones a woman in an *in vitro* treatment has been induced to "super ovulate," and she may have produced more eggs for fertilization than her uterus can cope with. Since uterine implantation is still the least successful step in *in vitro* treatments, most doctors implant four embryos in the hope that one or two will take. When there are embryos left over, should they be thrown away?

Asks Leon R. Kass, who is actively concerned with the ethical issues raised by the life sciences, "Who decides the grounds for discard? What if there is another recipient available who wishes to have the otherwise unwanted embryo? Whose embryos are they? The woman's? The couple's? The geneticist's? The obstetrician's? The Ford Foundation's? . . . Shall we say that discarding laboratory-grown embryos is a matter solely between a doctor and his plumber?"

Insists Dr. Hodgen at the Jones Institute emphatically, "We have not, we do not, and we will not create human embryos and discard them."

But many other clinics do create human embryos that will not be implanted. What happens to them?

Doctor Stillman prefers "to leave them in the laboratory until they stop growing. That will usually take a couple of days. We prefer not to take an active role in stopping their growth; we don't stop them, we just let them continue. Obviously there are strict limits on how long they can grow."

To people who believe that a person is created at conception, letting the embryos die is manslaughter, even though, as Stillman says, "We are talking about stopping growth at sixteen or thirty-two cells, still an extreme minimal small number of cells. Potential human life, absolutely, but very different than a baby in a test tube." Those not opposed to abortion cannot allow themselves to be morally upset if these tiny embryos are flushed down the toilet.

One way to get around the issue is to freeze the embryos. "Freezing will minimize the dilemma on one level," Stillman says, "but perhaps exacerbate it on many others."

In 1983 a rich American couple died in a plane crash. They left behind no offspring—or did they? The couple, who suffered from infertility, had enrolled in an *in vitro* clinic in Australia. They left two frozen embryos behind in Australia. What was to be done with the orphaned embryos after their death? Were they to be destroyed or implanted in a surrogate and given up for adoption? Did the embryos have a right to inherit their parents' $7 million estate? It all came down to a question of whether embryos are people or just a bunch of cells? No decision has been made yet because, as of this writing, the case is still lingering in court.

Dr. Jane Chihal, a reproductive endocrinologist in private practice in Dallas, Texas, puts only three embryos back into the womb and freezes all the rest. To avoid uncertainties about their fate, she asks the couples to decide what they want to happen to them and to make provisions for them in their will.

Freezing the embryos gives them another chance at life and saves both doctor and patient time, trouble, and money. If one transfer does not take, there is another embryo waiting in the nitrogen tank. Even if the first one leads to a full-term pregnancy, another embryo can be implanted later, so the first born gets a sibling that is his/her twin but born a year or more later.

Dr. DiMattina, who does a variation of *in vitro* called GIFT, admits, "We don't know what is the best number of eggs. I put four back because that is what most people are doing. But there is a person in London who is very famous—I won't mention names—he's putting back more than four. He will put back eight, and he has had a high incidence of multiple gestation—quadruplets, quintuplets, and so forth—and these have to be terminated as pregnancies. They don't have to be, but do you know how many quintuplets make it to term? Almost zero. So you're talking about death and prematurity.''

You are damned if you do not put all the embryos back, and you are damned if you do. With every new solution the stakes are upped.

"People who are faced with a multiple pregnancy, triplets and more, have elected to perform selective feticide." Dr. DiMattina explains as he continues the saga of what may happen when infertility is turned into superabundance. "A needle is placed through the abdominal wall into the uterine sac, and that sac is aspirated, thereby allowing one or two to hopefully survive rather than having three or four children. That has been done. Even if you eliminate GIFT and IVF and look at straight Pergonal, there are many—I shouldn't say many—instances where superovulatory multiple gestations have occurred and people have used selective feticide. You see, it is a crap shoot, isn't it?''

Dr. Fletcher thinks "selective termination of fetuses that are normal is offensive, but it is a kind of lifeboat situation. There is a tendency in infertility to get us into more of these lifeboat situations, which in the long run create a disrespect for human life. This is the kind of hazardous ethical life that you want to avoid.''

When Does Personhood Begin?

In cases of multiple gestations, not only the fate of the fetuses are on the line; the mother, too, is at both psychological and medical risk. However, in discussions about the ethics of IVF, it is the moral status of the embryo that takes center stage. Is it a person or simply a collection of a few cells?

There are many people who accord the embryo the full rights of a living member of society. If that view were enforced, *in vitro*, as it is being performed in most places, would be outlawed. But according the embryo full constitutional rights would have wider implications.

"If you follow that line of ethical reasoning," argues Dr. Fletcher, "then the social changes in the interest of justice and equality between men and women, which have been hard won, are going to be lost; the trend will be reversed. If a woman has to behave as if what she is carrying—even if it is only thirty seconds old—is a full-fledged person with the constitutional right to survive, it means that society is obligated to guard her during pregnancy. You can't have it both ways. If you start guarding women during pregnancy, it means that you have to keep them in some kind of captivity." And who comes out ahead in that situation? asks Dr. Fletcher. "Men."

The uncertain status of the fetus has made government take the cautious approach. It has refused to support *in vitro* research and, says Fletcher, "The consequences are terrible. The scientists suffer, and the parents suffer because they can't get accurate scientific information, and there is no peer review or judgment of what is good or bad in the field. The government has abdicated responsibility because it is politically unpopular with some voters."

A Biomedical Ethics Board established by Congress, consisting of six members from the House and six from the Senate will, with advice from an advisory board of scientists and ethicists, decide whether or not to lift the 1975 ban on fetal and embryo research. The moratorium on such research expires October 31, 1988. Some scientists feel held back and are concerned that research in the United States is falling behind while other countries make new discoveries. Australian researchers, for instance, have successfully fertilized a human egg by the injection of a single sperm. And in London, a clinic that will screen embryos for defects is scheduled to open.

At the moment the federal government may err on the side of caution, in the opinion of many scientists who, like Dr. Fletcher, think that brain activity determines the status of personhood.

"It means that at the end of life and at the beginning of life we are not persons," he argues. "When the brain is not yet there and when the brain is gone, you're not a person. Now, there are rituals of respect for the pre-person and the no-longer person, and these rituals ought to be preserved." But inasmuch as society finds it acceptable to remove organs from the body when the brain no longer functions, and since we do not consider a brain-dead human being a person, should we treat an organism that has not yet developed a brain as a person and forbid research on the embryo?

Human life indisputably begins when a woman's egg and a man's sperm fuse into one cell containing all the genetic information necessary to create a human being. That is how all vertebrate life starts. What distinguishes a human cell from those of other animals is the genetic information that tells it to grow into a human. As the cells undergo division, they pass through the same early stages as other vertebrates and are distinctly nonhuman in their characteristics. Said geneticist John Neel, "I cannot resist pointing out that quite early the embryo has gill slits and has an appendage labeled a tail in every textbook on embryology. Is it human at the time it is exhibiting gill slits and a tail?''[44]

Both church and state for a long time held the view that a fetus was not a person until it was animated by the ''rational soul,'' and both church and state permitted abortion until ''quickening.'' It was not until 1803 that Britain first passed antiabortion laws, and the United States followed suit in 1880. Even the Catholic Church's crusade against abortion is relatively recent. It started in 1869, when Pope Pius IV declared it to be murder.[45]

The definition of personhood is not a historical absolute. It depends on the society in which we live, and it changes not only with our medical knowledge but with our needs and our politics. It may not be entirely coincidental that the view of the fetus as a full human being was being advanced at the time of European expansionism, when more offspring were needed to carry ''the white man's burden,'' and when offspring were also needed to fuel industrialization and the taming of America. However, regardless of the motives, it may be argued that it did represent a raising of people's moral consciousness.

Have the technological skills that allow us to perform safe abortions and create disembodied embryos, which may then be discarded, cut up, and/or experimented upon, made us revert to old barbaric practices of feticide and disrespect for human life? Perhaps on some levels we have reverted. But science, as it advances, may well make pure nonsense of the position that the single cell created by an egg and a sperm is a person. The cell created by the fusion of an egg and a sperm is only human and distinguishable from a similar mammal cell insofar as it contains the genetic information necessary to develop a human being and not a bear. But every cell in our body, except the sex cells, contains all the information needed for any of our cells to grow into a human being. Scientists have already been able to create a frog from one frog body cell. They took a frog egg, removed the nucleus containing all the genetic information, and into the hollow egg they inserted a cell taken from the belly of another frog. The egg developed into a tadpole and ultimately into a frog. Scientists had cloned a frog. Cloning a human is not possible yet, but as soon as any cell in the body—blood cells, skin cells, muscle cells, or whatever—can be used to create a new human being (identical to the person from whom the cells were taken), are we then to save every drop of blood because it contain cells capable of becoming human life?

We run into absurdity if we maintain the position that every single cell that could grow into a person should be given full human rights. At the moment, people only consider the cell created at the moment of conception worthy of personhood status, but logically, once cloning becomes possible, we will have to extend the same rights to all cells. In a strange way, science and technology may well increase our respect for human life.

The Therapeutic Potential of External Fertilization

External fertilization is partly responsible for our changing perceptions and our confusion and our fears. Although, as Dr. Jane Chihal points out, *in vitro* "is becoming more popular as patients are realizing it is available to them, it is still on the bottom of the list" of reproductive options.

But Dr. Mark Geier of Genetics Consultants in Maryland foresees the day when people—if they had a choice in the matter—would choose to be conceived outside the body. Dr. Geier explains the projected advantages of having started life in a petri dish: "Supposing you could take the embryo at the eight-cell stage and remove a couple of cells, which I understand is being done with cattle—those cells, incidentally, would be identical twins. Supposing you froze them away, and the person grew up—the cells are in the freezer—and now the person gets to be fifty years old and has terminal heart disease. You take those cells out and you grow them in organ and tissue culture—you grow a new heart and give the person a heart and you give him another thirty years of life. No rejection—your heart, your cells. I think that's great."

That scenario is not right around the corner, but what to the layman seems nothing but a scientist's flight of fancy usually becomes living reality sooner or later, and scientists are already hard at work turning science fiction into mundane medical treatments.

The ability to grow embryos outside the womb holds the promise of eliminating genetic defects. Because the embryo is outside the body and can be studied, manipulated, and perhaps tampered with, *in vitro* has opened up the possibility of eliminating inherited diseases. *In vitro* conception has made some forms of intervention "absolutely easier," says Dr. Fletcher. "Disease could be fixed in the embryo." Scientists are now learning to determine the sex of the embryo and, says Fletcher, "In certain suspected sex-linked genetic diseases, like muscular dystrophy, you will be able to put all male embryos aside and only implant the female. That's a great step unless you think that putting those aside is the moral equivalent of abortion. The ultimate fix would be in the sperm and egg cells, if you could figure out a way to transform these gametes without killing them. I'm sure that's where it's going to go.''

At the moment, using an assortment of prenatal tests, it is possible to detect about 560 genetic diseases while the baby is still in the womb. A few afflictions, like spina bifida, a neural tube defect, may soon be treated surgically in the womb.

"They do a sort of C-section," explains Mark Geier. "They open up the uterus, take the baby out, and do surgery for spinal defects. They don't detach the placenta, they don't detach the cord, put the baby back in, sew the mother up. The only reason to think you can't do that is that the mother would go into labor, but now we have drugs to stop labor.''

Such surgical experiments have been done on monkeys and, says Dr. Geier, "the monkeys do fine, and I have every reason to believe that humans would, too.''

But for a host of other genetic diseases, the only "treatment" is abortion and, as Dr. Geier says, to most parents, especially those who have suffered from infertility, "abortion is catastrophic. No one wants to abort. We all want to treat.''

". . . In the United States and Britain, genetic disorders are known to occur in between three and five percent of all live births, and chromosomal disorders—for example, Down's syndrome—in at least one-half percent. The percentages may be small, but the absolute annual numbers suggest a wrenching magnitude of individual afflictions—in the United States, up to one hundred and sixty-five thousand abnormal infants, including from six to eight thousand with neural tube defects like spina bifida, five thousand cases of Down's syndrome, fifteen hundred of cystic fibrosis, at least a thousand of sickle-cell anemia. Genetic and chromosomal illnesses or malformations are reported to account for between twenty and thirty percent of all pediatric hospital admissions. Twelve percent of all adult hospital admissions are said to involve illnesses with a significant genetic component. At least fifteen percent of all diagnoses for mental retardation report it as unambiguously hereditary.''[46]

Although it is very hard to isolate the specific functions of individual genes, which are responsible for everything from hair color to retardation, researchers have succeeded in identifying, for example, the precise gene defect that causes one out of every 2,000 babies to be born with cystic fibrosis. Genes are located at specific sites on specific chromosomes, and scientists are now learning to locate and map out the gene geography. The mapping process began in the early 1970s, and today more than 800 human genes have been located on the chromosomes. Eventually we will know exactly what traits each gene is responsible for and where to find them, so that if an embryo has a defective gene, it can be replaced by a "good" one. And since genes are inherited, future generations would also be spared the possibility of being afflicted by the disease. The technical capability, however, is not yet available.

"Right now we do not have the ability to splice in a new gene where the old defective one was and kick the old one out," cautions Dr. Evelyn Karson, a senior staff fellow at the National Institutes of Health. "I want to make that one clear—it is not like videotape splicing. It is not to say that it might not eventually be." And *in vitro* conception has made that eventuality less utopian.

It is already possible to screen for a few genes if you know what you are looking for.

"It is technically feasible," says Dr. Karson, "to take an egg and sperm and fertilize *in vitro* and wait till it divides to eight cells. You take the eight cells, separate them into eight parts, you freeze each one, then take one, grow it up to eight cells, and so on. So it is possible to detect a single gene. The problem is you can't do that for every single gene. You're limited by the amount of samples you can safely get without destroying the organism. But it will be feasible to take an embryo cell and look for a single gene to see if it is normal or not."

Says Dr. Gary Hodgen, "We are going be applying IVF to a wider spectrum of medical problems, such as preventing birth defects. [We will] look at the gene structure to see if the embryos are normal or not." And these diagnostic techniques will eventually be used on embryos of people who can conceive normally. "These people are not infertile, they want a well child," says Hodgen.

We would probably all like to eliminate genetic diseases, but few of us would like geneticists to design humans according to government standards. When we read that scientists have already created animals that never set foot in Noah's ark, we become uncomfortable. Genetic engineers have produced gigantic pigs, and a whole new patented creation, the geep, a cross between a goat and a sheep. If we can improve or create bigger and better and even new animals, can humans be far behind?

Yes, says Evelyn Karson, because "it is sort of an unwritten law now that human gene therapy will only be done on the somatic cells [those not involved in reproduction]. I would like to know a little more about the somatic cells before we start messing with one that is going to be passed on, because if we create something that is a mistake, there is going to be a problem.''

Evelyn Karson, pregnant at the time we spoke with her, is not worried about messing with the essence of humanity.

"We are not doing anything right now that might not have happened on its own. We are acting as catalysts so that the rate at which these changes occur may be more rapid. But I guess I have a certain faith in the concept of natural selection, and I'm not sure there was some single preordained path.''

She is also not sure whether "technology is the symptom of change or the mover of change,'' but says, "I have grown up with things changing. I'm not afraid of that. I'm just old enough now to be completely awed by the changes that have gone on in science. I look at all these DNA techniques. There was almost nothing when I was in graduate school from 1972 to 1977.'' She is convinced the speed of change is going to increase because "you're talking about logarithmic progression.''

Although many people are afraid, there does not seem to be a way of stopping developments, and should we if it means that a lot of presently incurable diseases could be eliminated?

Mark Geier sees the same ultimate benefits from genetic treatments as we have seen from more sophisticated delivery techniques and technology.

"Until say twenty years ago, obstetrics concentrated primarily on eliminating damage due to lack of oxygen at birth. If you went to the institutions in the old days, most of them were filled with people who were damaged at birth—cerebral palsy and that kind of thing. Now we are very good at this; there are very few babies damaged that way. Now if you look at institutions, the main thing you'll see are genetic disorders, and they are not insignificant. They represent three to five percent of all babies born, and it accounts for [a large] percent of our health care dollars to take care of these children.''

If man could fix some of God's mistakes, shouldn't we go right ahead? Geier thinks so: "The obvious benefits are so powerful that it is not a choice; it is something that's going to happen. When there are obvious benefits for things that we absolutely need, people are going to develop them, and I think that every mother wants to give life to a normal child.''

The Quest for Perfect Children

"Couples now have only one or two children, and there is no question they demand perfection, but they have unrealistic expectations of us," says Dr. Maurice Druzin, director of obstetrics at New York Hospital. "The public doesn't understand that there are things over which we have no control."[47]

Just as this generation makes decisions based on a chart—advantages on one side and disadvantages on the other—just as it does not buy anything without checking *Consumer Reports* for its recommendation or go to a restaurant without a review, this generation approaches childbearing with all the options in mind. We want to have the best available child for our money.

The ideal child is one that lives up to our expectations. If at all possible, it has to be our own, and preferably of the "right" sex.

A company called ProCare made money off $49.95 "Gender Choice" kits that were supposed to help prospective parents select the sex of their child before conception. The kit, containing disposable thermometers, materials for sampling vaginal mucus, and instructions, was based on a theory that female-producing sperm may be more likely to reach the egg just when ovulation takes place, while male-producing sperm may be more likely to succeed shortly after ovulation. On January 21, 1987, the FDA declared Gender Choice "a gross deception of the consumer."[48] It was a trivial attempt to create the boy or girl envisioned and only hurt people's pocketbooks, but the wish to select the sex of a child has in some cases turned amniocentesis, which reveals the gender of the fetus, from a diagnostic test into a death sentence. If the child is not the right sex, it is aborted.

Few people would condone carrying demands for perfection to such frivolous and fatal lengths, but there are many situations where the choice between giving birth and aborting is not morally simple. Mild retardation—not painful or crippling except to parents who hope for a super baby—is less and less accepted. Then there are situations where the defects are so serious as to make life a painful experience, where for the sake of the child and the parents abortion seems more merciful. In the past there was no way of knowing before birth if the fetus had congenital defects; now we expect the doctors to warn us.

In 1978 a couple from Long Island, New York, the Beckers, brought suit against their obstetrician. Dolores Becker had become pregnant at the age of thirty-seven and had given birth to a girl with Down's syndrome. According to the Beckers' complaint, their doctor had not warned them of the higher incidence of

Down's syndrome in children born to mothers over thirty-five and had not offered to perform amniocentesis, which would have indicated that the child would be born retarded. Not only did the Beckers want the obstetrician held financially accountable for the cost of caring for their daughter, they also wanted him held accountable for "wrongful causation of life," on the grounds that their daughter had been denied the "fundamental right of a child to be born as a whole, functional human being." The New York State Court of Appeals, however, disallowed the second claim as a basis for suit, holding that "whether it is better to have been born at all than to have been born with even gross deficiencies is a mystery more properly left to the philosophers and the theologians."[49]

The California State Court of Appeals was not daunted by divine mysteries in 1980, when it ruled on a "wrongful life" action brought by Temar Curlander on behalf of his daughter Shauna. Curlander and his wife had consulted the Bio-Science and Automated Laboratory Sciences in 1977 to determine whether either of them carried the recessive gene for Tay-Sachs disease, caused by an enzyme deficiency that can lead to blindness and invariably to an early death, usually around the age of four. The hereditary disease most often affects Jews. The laboratory tests showed that the Curlanders had nothing to fear, but when Shauna was born she was diagnosed as a Tay-Sachs baby. Her parents sued the labs for compensation for the suffering endured during her expected four-year life-span and for having been deprived of 72.6 years of normal life. The courts disallowed the normal life-span argument but did allow the Curlanders "to recover damages for the pain and suffering." Explained the court, "The reality of the 'wrongful life' concept is that such a plaintiff both exists and suffers, due to the negligence of others. It is neither necessary nor just to retreat into meditation on the mysteries of life. . . . The certainty of genetic impairment is no longer a mystery."[50]

Whether it was right or wrong for these children to be born comes down, in the words of Kennedy Institute ethicist Abigail Evans, to whether "you deem physical life in and of itself more important than the quality of life." In these cases the quality of life may have been so poor as to be virtually no life at all. But what is significant about these cases is a fundamental change in our view of life. We no longer just demand to have children when we want them and how we want them, we demand that they be healthy children.

Any normal parents hope to have a sound child, but says Daniel Callahan of the Hastings Center, "We will indeed have descended into the pit if we make genetic perfection a condition for the right to exist."[51]

The right of only the perfect to exist is not yet public policy, but every time a doctor aborts a fetus that he has diagnosed as abnormal, we are in effect operating on that principle. And there are voices calling for laws that would mandate abortions of defective fetuses.

According to attorney Mary Sue Henifin, "Some legal commentators do not think that a pregnant woman has the right to refuse prenatal diagnosis or the right to carry a pregnancy to term if she knows that the fetus has a genetic defect." She notes that "jurist Marjory Shaw has stated that a woman who decides 'to carry a genetically fetus to term' should incur liability fetal abuse."[52]

While most people would encourage the possibilities of eliminating genetic disease, preferably by treatment, few of us would like the government to set standards of human perfection.

Crippling diseases of the mind and of the body cause enormous suffering to both the children and their parents. In the past such tragedies were seen as a blow dealt by "unkind fate," but today many congenital afflictions are blamed on the technicians. High expectations were cited in a recent American Medical Association report as a key reason why obstetricians are the most-sued physicians in the United States. We want and expect a perfect child to come out of the medical workshop. The sick children that slip through the screening have, we say, been given "wrongful life," a concept that has meaning only in a society where technology has given us choices in an area where there were never any choices before. Not only do we want the technicians to assume responsibility, we want a money back guarantee. We are inching towards the view of children as manufactured goods.

"We have these things around us that are perfect," says a forty-year-old man who offered to be a sperm donor. "You buy something and it's just like the one next to it, which is just like ones in the other store. It's a natural next step to expect that of our bodies. For the most part, our lives revolve around machine-made things. It takes a thinking person to realize that you can't expect of life what you can of your Toyota."

The pressure is on to have perfect children—from conception to adulthood. What started with contraception and the wish to have only wanted children has become a demand that the child we want be perfect.

Couples contemplating a surrogate baby quite understandably shop around for good I.Q. scores and look at photos to find the best-looking potential surrogate; *in vitro* parents will soon be able to screen the embryo for defects before it is implanted; and all of us can have a fetus in the womb tested. If the baby to be delivered is not up to our expectations, we can cancel the order.

This consumer attitude to procreation is a phenomenon that writer Richard Cohen has dubbed "procreative capitalism."

"Some people want a child that is theirs, that in some sense they own. It is as if they seek to clone themselves and then treat the child as an extension of themselves—a statement of who they are. In this sense, children become consumer goods, like cars. They announce status. For some the perfect child is one who behaves the way they would like, attends the 'right' schools and then has a career that complements those of the parents. . . ."[53]

Neither conception nor child rearing is done by instinct any longer. Parenthood is something couples study for if they want that desired super baby. Using the latest nutritional information, they prime their bodies before conception and during pregnancy; they learn breathing techniques in Lamaze classes; and when the baby is born, they enrich its environment in the crib and on every step through childhood.

At the Better Baby Institute in Philadelphia, founder Glen Doman offers classes to parents so they can teach their babies to recognize a Picasso painting. Books such as Eric Johnson's *Raising Children to Achieve,* Muriel Schoenbrun Karlin's *Making Your Child a Success*, and *How to Maximize Your Child's Potential* are among the guides available for parents who want perfect children.

"Many mothers and fathers have turned parenthood into a painfully competitive sport," says Martha Weinman Lear. "In an era when traditional status symbols can turn obsolescent overnight, they have discovered that social stature may still be gained by raising the best-dressed, -fed, -educated, -mannered, -medicated, -cultured, and -adjusted child on the block."[54]

"Somehow children of upper income families are seen as an extension of one's success," says Constance Shapiro. "Children are not being valued for who they are, only for what they can bring their parents in way of credit, or recognition. I can only wonder if it has something to do with the keeping-up-with-the-Joneses phenomenon in the fifties to the eighties, where one's children are seen just as the boat and the extra car in the garage—as one more notch in the belt of accomplishment that is better than one's peers and one's neighbors."

A New View of Childhood

For better or worse, our views of children and childhood have changed radically, to a large extent due to advances in our knowledge and medical capabilities.

Philip Aries, in *Centuries of Childhood*, shows that our modern idea of children is much different from what it used to be. Childhood, unlike its status today, was merely a place people passed through on their way to adulthood.

"The child . . . was not missing from the Middle Ages . . . but there was never a portrait of him, the portrait of a real child, as he was at a certain moment of his life. The general feeling was, and for a long time remained, that one had several children in order to keep just a few. People could not allow themselves to become too attached to something that was regarded as a probable loss . . . the child that had died too soon in life was buried almost anywhere, much as we today bury a domestic pet, a cat or a dog. He was such an unimportant little thing, so inadequately involved in life.[55]

"Nobody thought, as we ordinarily think today," writes Aries, "that every child already contained a man's personality."[56]

Today we take childhood seriously from the word *go*. The baby is kept close to the mother with soft lights and comforting temperatures and pleasant music. The revolution in baby bearing is both hard and soft. At the same time that we use *in vitro* fertilization, we are more concerned with maternal bonding. On the one hand we abort defective fetuses, on the other, we treat those created by extraordinary means with increased respect.

"An odd thing is happening," says Fletcher. "At the same time as we are selectively going in and killing fetuses, the moral status of the fetus is increasing in society because of all the things you can do, but mainly because you can see it at a very early time."

Today many baby books do not start with photographs of the wrinkly newborn but with sonographic pictures of the child as a fetus. Some *in vitro* parents even have a photograph of their child as an eight-cell embryo. And the famous pictorial history by Swedish photographer Lennart Nielson, now a Time-Life book, of the development of the fetus in the womb—the fetus sprouting fingers and toes, the fetus sucking its thumb—make us relate to the "thing" behind a woman's abdominal wall in a more emotional and personal way.

"Bonding increases much earlier, and we are generating a new stage of life, fetal, which, I believe will be as real to our children and grandchildren as childhood is today," says Fletcher. "Childhood was really not an authentic stage of life until the twentieth century. We didn't understand children, nor did we give them a life of their own. They were projections. The fetus will undergo the same evolution.''

On the Horns of New Dilemmas

The new ways of creating babies have in many ways caught us in a number of contradictions. We strive to create high-tech babies, and in the next room we perform abortions on demand. We consider bonding very important, while at the same time we contract with surrogates for babies to be given away. We do not want to associate babies with money, but we happily pay physicians, surrogates, and agencies large sums to create them. We are caught in a web of warring attitudes, motivations, and ethics.

The only person who can make us momentarily overcome all these contradictions gives no advice and holds no views on these matters. It is the baby. The baby ultimately makes us captives not of doctors, not of theorists, lawyers, psychologists, or other experts, but of our own emotions, which—when it comes to babies—are luckily totally incomprehensible. We love babies unconditionally once they are there.

''When my firstborn daughter was six weeks old we went to the pediatrician with her for the usual scheduled visit. . . . My general impression as a scientist—that newborn babies all looked the same and were quite unappealing . . . was confirmed for me by my experience as a father,'' writes anthropologist Melvin Konner.

''I held the baby up to the light, squinted at the physician out of one bloodshot eye, and made my statement starkly and clearly: 'Tell me, Doctor,' I said, 'You've been in this business for a long time. (I now glanced meaningfully at the baby.) 'She's ruining my life. She's ruining my sleep, she's ruining my health, she's ruining my work, she's ruining my relationship with my wife, and . . . and . . . and she's ugly . . . why do I like her?'

''The physician, a distinguished one in our town, and a wise and old and a virtuous man, seemed most unbaffled by the problem.

'' 'You know'—he shrugged his shoulders—'parenting is an instinct and the baby is the releaser.' ''[57]

Epilogue

IN JULY 1987 THE WORLD POPULATION PASSED THE 5 BILLION mark.

While global concerns concentrate on reducing the number of people in the world, a small number of infertility doctors and scientists are coming up with new ways of adding members to the human race.

How, in a world that undeniably suffers from too many people, can we justify the resource expenditure and the "selfishness" of making miracle babies?

It is not a question that infertile—or for that matter fertile—couples agonize over when they decide to have children. In fact, there often seems to be what Alice Taylor Day calls "the gap between private behavior and pubic needs."

"Demographic history," she writes, "has demonstrated repeatedly that the family-building habits of couples are almost totally uninfluenced by demographic considerations. In European countries the biggest advances in the spread of family limitation came in the 20s and the 30s against a background of official alarm about the possibility of underpopulation. During the 1960s, in many of these same countries, the three-or-four-child family was gain-

275

ing in popularity, particularly among certain higher socio-economic groups, and this time at a time of increasing public concern with the threat of overpopulation."[1]

While attempts to create miracle babies may seem irresponsible to some, the number of children created in extraordinary ways is not large enough to set off even a small population explosion. Perhaps 20,000 or more people in the world today are the result of donor insemination, about 5,000 have entered the world through IVF or related techniques, and another 600 or more are surrogate children.

If these children are unnecessary from a demographic standpoint, IVF babies, at least, may have contributed to the world in ways that will benefit everybody. Just as progress in some scientific research that does not seem to bear any relation to general human needs—the space program, for instance—often brings us unforeseen benefits, "advances in reproductive technologies have repercussions far beyond the first line issues," says Norfolk's Gary Hodgen. He believes that the very basic egg-and-sperm research that led to the development of IVF will take us beyond fullfilling the wishes of infertile couples.

External fertilization grew out of research into contraception, and now IVF may in turn lead to better and safer birth control. Dr. Hodgen believes that new studies on the receptivity of egg to sperm will lead to a vaccine for both men and women that would prevent egg and sperm from fusing—a technical advance that may reduce teenage pregnancies, reduce the need for abortions, and better stem the world's population growth.

But of even greater benefit to mankind may be the insight that the embryo in a petri dish has given us into the growth of cells. By learning about the mechanics of cell growth, scientist may eventually find a cure for cancer.

"By studying the human embryonic cells in the lab, I believe the chance is the highest of any approach to understanding what the new treatment of cancer will be," says Hodgen. "Early in the twenty-first century, there will be methods of cancer therapy based not on surgery, not on chemotherapy, not on irradiation, but on turning off the function of the cell that's causing the tumor to grow. I think we can learn how to do that by studying normal embryonic cells."

However, scientific advances are not just a question of science but of politics. At the moment, U.S. laws severely restrict the opportunity to study human embryonic cell growth, and it is a touchy topic not popular with Right-to-Life activists and other voters.

"Politics always exists where there is less than a consensus," says Hodgen. "If you have a consensus, there's no political point of view." Since there is little consensus on the subject of making babies in new ways, "it is a political agenda and will remain so," Hodgen predicts.

Society needs to digest and interpret—but quickly—the new social and scientific ideas in the context of our culture, goals, and priorities, and ultimately our own humanness. Both the dangers and benefits of new methods of conception are great, and both are difficult to predict accurately. As one scientist explained by way of analogy, "The guy who invented the wheel invented a great thing, but it had a lot of uses he didn't foresee. He might have been rather dismayed to see it on a B-52 bomber." But, says the same scientist, that is no reason for stopping, for "it is never technology that is evil, it is only what man does with it that may be."

New ways of making babies have the potential for increasing the sum of human happiness, but in order to avoid abuses, we need to set limits and goals for the social and scientific spin-offs of our own procreative inventiveness.

Bibliography

Although we have not written a consumer book for infertile couples who want to get pregnant, many authors have. For couples in search of this kind of information, there are many excellent reference books available which will guide you to the right doctor, the right clinic, or the right lawyer. Those marked with an * will provide good resource material.

Achilles, Rona Grace, *The Social Meanings of Biological Ties: A Study of Participants in Artificial Insemination by Donor*. University of Toronto Doctoral Dissertation, 1986.

*Andrews, Lori B., *New Conceptions: A Consumer's Guide to the Newest Infertility Treatments*, Ballantine Books. New York, 1984.

Ariès, Philippe, *Centuries of Childhood: A Social History of Family Life*. Vintage Books, New York, 1962.

Bellina, Joseph H., and Wilson, Josleen, *You Can Have a Baby*. New York, Bantam Books, 1986.

Berman, Phyllis W., and Ramey, Estelle R., eds., *Women: A Developmental Perspective*. U.S. Department of Health and Human Services, National Institutes of Health, 1982.

Boston Women's Health Book Collective, *The New Our Bodies, Ourselves*, Simon & Schuster. New York, 1984.

Corea, Gena. *The Mother Machine: Reproductive Technologies from Artificial Insemination to Artificial Wombs*. Harper & Row, New York, 1985.

Curto, Josephine J. *How to Become a Single Parent: A Guide for Single People Considering Adoption or Natural Parenthood Alone.* Prentice-Hall, Inc., Englewood Cliffs, New Jersey, 1983.

Edwards, Robert and Steptoe, Patrick. *A Matter of Life: The Story of a Medical Breakthrough.* William Morrow and Company, Inc., New York, 1980.

Greer, Germaine, *Sex and Destiny: Politics of Human Fertility.* Harper & Row, New York, 1984.

Grobstein, Clifford. *From Chance to Purpose: An Appraisal of External Human Fertilization.* Addison-Wesley Publishing Company, Reading, Massachusetts, 1981.

Keane, Noel P. with Breo, Dennis L. *The Surrogate Mother.* Everest House Publishers, New York, 1981.

Kevles, Daniel J. *In the Name of Eugenics.* University of California Press, 1985.

Kirkendall, Lester A., and Whitehurst, Robert, eds., *The New Sexual Revolution.* Donald W. Brown, Inc., New York, 1971.

Means, Cyril C., Jr. "Surrogacy v. The Thirteenth Amendment," *The New York Law School Human Rights Annual.* Volume IV, Issue 2, 1987.

*Menning, Barbara Eck, *Infertility: A Guide for Childless Couples.* Prentice-Hall, New Jersey, 1977.

*Perloe, Mark and Christie, Linda Gail. *Miracle Babies & Other Happy Endings for Couples with Fertility Problems.* Rawson Associates, New York, 1986.

Robinson, L. Susan, *Having a Baby Without a Man* Simon & Schuster, New York, 1985.

Salzer, Linda, *Infertility: How Couples Can Cope.* Boston, G. K. Hall & Co., 1986.

*Silver, Sherman J. *How to Get Pregnant.* Warner Books, New York, 1980.

Singer, Peter, and Wells, Deane, *Making Babies: The New Science and Ethics of Conception.* Charles Scribner's Sons, New York, 1984.

*Tilton, Nan and Todd & Gaylen Moore, *Making Miracles: In Vitro Fertilization.* Doubleday, New York, 1985.

Notes

CHAPTER 1 Why Children?

1. Mark Jacobsen, "The Baby Chase", *Esquire* May 1987.
2. Barbara Eck Menning, *Infertility: A Guide for Childless Couples* Prentice-Hall, New Jersey, 1977, p. 111.
3. Ibid., p. 108.
4. Linda Salzer, *Infertility: How Couples Can Cope*. Boston, G.K. Hall & Co., 1986. p. 24.
5. "Three's a Crowd," *Newsweek*, September 1, 1986.
6. Ibid.
7. Madeleine Blais, "Why Have Children?" *Washington Post Magazine*, May 9, 1982.
8. Stephen A. Richardson and Alan Gluttmacher, eds., *Childbearing: It's Social and Psychological Aspects* (Baltimore, 1967) quoted in Germaine Greer, *Sex and Destiny: The Politics of Human Fertility*, p. 47.
9. Richard Cohen, "A Child of One's Own" *Washington Post Magazine*, February 15, 1987.
10. *Newsweek*, op cit.

11. Menning, p. 120.

12. Greer, p.

13. *Newsweek*, op cit.

14. Greer, p. 39.

15. *Newsweek*, op cit.

16. Gael Greene quoted in Martha Weinman Lear, *The Child Worshippers*, New York, Crown Publishers, Inc., 1963.

17. Hamed Ammar, *Growing Up*, quoted in Greer, op. cit., p. 61.

18. V. Ebin, "Interpretations of Infertility and Birth: The Aowin of Western Ghana," in *Ethnography of Fertility and Birth*, edited by C. P. MacCormack, London, 1982.

19. Bernie Zilbergeld, *The Shrinking of America: Myths of Psychological Change*. Little, Brown and Company, Boston, 1983, p. 40.

CHAPTER 2 Donor Insemination

1. J.K. Sherman, "Current Status of Clinical Cryobanking of Human Semen", in *Andrology: Male Fertility and Sterility*, Orlando, Academic Press, Inc., p. 534.

2. Sherman J. Silber, *How To Get Pregnant* New York: Warner Books, 1980, p. 1984.

3. Ibid, p. 179.

4. Lori Andrews, *New Conceptions: A Consumer's Guide to the Newest Infertility*, New York: Ballantine Books, 1984, p. 148.

5. Silber, op. cit., p. 180.

6. Gena Corea, *The Mother Machine: Reproductive Technologies from Artificial Insemination to Artificial wombs*, New York: Harper & Row, 1985, p. 34.

7. Rona Grace Achilles, *The Social Meanings of Biological Ties: A Study of Participants in Artificial Insemination by Donor*, University of Toronto Doctoral Dissertation, 1986, p. 46.

8. "Declaration on Certain Questions Concerning Sexual Ethics", DSP pamphlet, p. 14.

9. "A Rush of Test-Tube Babies Ahead?," *U.S. News & World Report*, August 7, 1978.

10. Achilles, op. cit., p. 126.

11. Silber, op. cit., p. 173.

12. Achilles, op. cit., p. 11.

13. Ibid.

14. Ibid.

15. Ibid., p. 71.

16. Ibid.

17. Ibid., p. 76.

18. Ibid., p. 67.
19. ibid., p. 69.
20. Ibid.
21. Ibid., p. 62.
22. Ibid., p. 69.
23. Andrews, p. 34.
24. Achilles, op. cit., p. 50.
25. Ibid., p. 130.
26. Ibid., p. 146.
27. Joseph Blizzard. *Blizzard and the Holy Ghost*, Peter Owen Ltd., London, 1977. (Exerpted by Donor's offspring)
28. Ibid.
29. Achilles, op. cit., p. 145.
30. Ibid.
31. Obituary, *New York Times*, January 28, 1984.
32. Joseph Bellina, and Josleen Wilson, *You Can Have a Baby* New York, Bantam Books, 1986, page 71.
33. Sherman, op. cit., p. 155.
34. Andrews, op. cit., p. 155.
35. Ibid.
36. Timothy J. McNulty, "High-Tech Motherhood Creates Social Rifts," *Chicago Tribune*, July 26, 1987.
37. *Congressoinal Quarterly*, April 29, 1983.
38. *American Journal of Obstetrics and Gynecology*, September 1986.
39. Mark and Christie Perloe, *Miracle Babies & Other Happy Endings for Couples with Fertility Problems*, edited by Linda Gail, Rawson Associates, New York, 1986, p. 229.
40. Sherman, op. cit., p. 532.
41. Andrews, op. cit., p. 150.
42. Andrews, op. cit., p. 173.
43. *Congressional Quarterly*, April 1983.
44. Corea, op. cit., p. 50.
45. Silber, p. 174.
46. Timothy J. McNulty, "Dilemma is born: Donor's rights vs. children's," *Chicago Tribune*, August 10, 1987.
47. Achilles, op. cit., p. 73.
48. Robin Rowland, "Attitudes and Opinions of Donors on an Artificial Insemination by Donor Programme." *Clinical Reproduction and Fertility*, February, 1983.
49. Achilles, op. cit., p. 7.
50. McNulty, op. cit., August 10, 1987.
51. Ibid.
52. Achilles, op. cit., p. 62.
53. Ibid., p. 136.

54. Ibid., p. 140.
55. Ibid., p. 138.
56. Ibid., p. 137.
57. McNulty, op. cit., August 10, 1987.
58. Dr. Robert Snowden and G. D. Mitchell, *The Artificial Family*, London, 1981. (excerpted by Donor's Offspring.)
59. Achilles, op. cit., p. 64.
60. Ibid., p. 9.

CHAPTER 3, In Vitro Fertilization

1. Linda Salzer, *Infertility: How Couples Can Cope*. Boston, G.K. Hall & Co., p. 19.
2. Ibid., p. 46.
3. Joseph H. Bellina and Josleen Wilson, *You Can Have a Baby*. New York, Bantam Books, 1986., p. 7.
4. Ibid., p. 237.
5. Lynda Stephenson, *Give Us a Child*, New York, Harper & Row, 1987. Quoted in Mary Hickey "The Quiet Pain of Infertility", Washington Post, April 28, 1987.
6. Salzer, op. cit., pp. 101–102.
7. Bellina and Wilson, op cit., p. 97.
8. Ibid., p. 167.

CHAPTER 4 Test Tube Babies

1. Robert Edwards and Patrick Steptoe, *A Matter of Life: The Story of a Medical Breakthrough*, New York, William Morrow and Company, Inc., 1980. p. 28.
2. Ibid., p. 30.
3. Ibid., p. 40.
4. Ibid., p. 45.
5. Ibid., p. 59.
6. Ibid., p. 60.
7. Ibid., p. 65.
8. Ibid., p. 80.
9. Ibid.
10. Tilton Nantood, and Gaylen Moore, *Making Miracles*: In Vitro fertilization. New York, Doubleday, 1985, p. 101–102.
11. Ibid., p. 113–114.
12. Ibid., p. 67.

13. Doug Brown, "Childless Couples. See New Hope: 'In Vitro', Los Angeles Times, October 6, 1985.
14. Linda P. Salzer, Infertility: How Couples Can Cope, Boston, G.K. Hall & Company, 1986, p. 135.

CHAPTER 5: Science Creates a New Business

1. Sandra Blakeslee, "Trying to Make Money Making 'Test Tube' Babies. *New York Times*, May 17, 1987.
2. Ibid.
3. Ibid.
4. Ibid.
5. Ibid.
6. Sandra Blakeslee, "Some Caveats for Childless Couples, *New York Times*, May 4, 1987.
7. Joseph H. Bellina and Josleen Wilson, *You Can Have a Baby*. New York, Bantam Books, 1986, p. 383.
8. Blakeslee, 1987. op. cit.
9. Blakeslee, 1986, op. cit.
10. Ibid.
11. Gena Corea, *The Mother Machine: Reproductive Technologies from Artificial Insemination to Artificial Wombs*, Harper & Row, 1985, p. 179.
12. Giovanna Breu and Mark Feldinger, "In California a small bundle of medical history arrives on time: the first frozen U.S. embryo baby." *People*, June 23, 1986.
13. Ibid.
14. Peter Singer & Dean Wells: *Making Babies: The New Science and Ethics of Conception* New York, Scribner & Sons, 1985, p. 33.
15. Corea, op. cit., p. 80.
16. Ibid., p. 95.
17. Corea, op. cit., p. 84.
18. Harris Brotman, "Human Embryo Transplants," *New York Times*, January 8, 1984.
19. Ibid.
20. Corea, op. cit., p. 86.
21. Brotman, op. cit.
22. Corea, op. cit., p. 85.
23. Ibid. p. 88.
24. Brotman, op. cit.
25. Timothy McNulty, "Growing Pains Afflict Birth Technology," *Chicago Tribune*, July 28, 1987.
26. Corea, op. cit., p. 85.

CHAPTER 6 Surrogacy

1. Ruth Marcus, "Baby M Fight goads legislatures" *Washington Post*, March 31, 1987.
2. Mark Rust: "Whose Baby is it?" *ABA Journal*, June 1987.
3. John Robertson, "At Issue" *ABA Journal*, June 1, 1987.
4. Lori Andrews, *New Conceptions: A Consumer's Guide to the Newest Infertility*, New York, Ballantine Books, 1984, p. 190.
5. Elizabeth Bumiller, "Mother for Others," *Washington Post*, March 9, 1983.
6. Andrews, p. 190.
7. Andrews, op. cit., p. 201.

CHAPTER 7 The Women Who Serve as Surrogates

1. Lori Andrews, *New Conceptions: A Consumer's Guide to the Newest Infertility*, New York, Ballantine Books, 1984, p. 196.
2. Noel Keane with Dennis Breo, *The Surrogate Mother*. New York, Everest House Publishers, 1981, pp. 227–228.
3. Andrews, op. cit. p. 202.
4. Keane, op. cit., 124.
5. Iver Peterson, "Surrogate Mothers Vent Feelings of Doubt and Joy," New York Times, March 2, 1987.
6. Ibid.
7. Lori Andrews. Testimony before the Select Committe on Children, Youth and Families", May 21, 1987.
8. Patricia Avery, "Surrogate Mothers: Center of a New Storm," U.S. News and World Reports, June 6, 1983.
9. David Behrens, "She Just Liked Being Pregnant," New York Newsday, January 13, 1987.
10. Michael Kinsley, "Baby M and the Moral Logic of Capitalism" Wall Street Journal, April 16, 1987.
11. Gena Corea, The Mother Machine: Reproductive Technologies from Artificial Insemination to Artificial Wombs. New York Harper & Row 1985, p. 229.
12. Barbara Katz Rothman, "Cheap Labor. Sex, Class, Race and Surrogacy" Unpublished paper.
13. George Wilder, Wealth and Poverty, New York, Basic Books, 1981, p. 9.
14. Ibid., pp. 24–25.
15. Ibid. p. 24.
16. Ibid. p. 25.

17. Elizabeth Bumiller, "Mothers for Others", Washington Post, March 9, 1983.
18. Ibid.
19. Mary Gordon, "Baby M: New Questions about Biology and Destiny", Ms. Magazine, June 1987.
20. Anne Taylor Fleming, "Our Fascination with Baby M", New York Times Magazine, March 29, 1987.

CHAPTER 9 The Moral and Ethical Issues of New Reproductive Technologies

1. John Robertson, "Testimony Before The Select Committee on Children, Youth and Family," Washington, D.C. May 21, 1987.
2. Sidney Callahan, "Lovemaking and Babymaking," *Commonweal*, April 2, 1987.
3. The Ethics Committee of the American Fertility Society, "Ethical Considerations of the New Reproductive Technologies," *Fertility and Sterility, Supplement 1*, September 1986, Vol. 45, No. 3.
4. Robert Marshall, "Testimony Before The Select Committee on Children, Youth and Family," Washington, D.C., May 21, 1987.
5. Susan Robinson, *Having a Baby Without a Man*, New York, Simon & Schuster, 1985, p. 23.
6. Gena Corea, *The Mother Machine: Reproductive Technologies from Artificial Insemination to Artificial Wombs*. New York, Harper & Row, 1985, p. 43.
7. Bernard Gore and Barbara Raboy, "Sperm Bank of Northern California, "Three Year Report: October 5, 1982–September 30, 1985.
8. Lester Kirkendall and Robert Whitehurst, eds., *The New Sexual Revolution*, New York, Donald W. Brown, Inc., New York, 1971, p. 115.
9. Corea, op. cit., p. 43.
10. Rona Grace Achilles, *The Social Meanings of Biological Ties: A Study of Participants in Artificial Insemination by Donor*, University of Toronto Doctoral Dissertation 1986, p. 41.
11. Ibid., p. 41.
12. Robinson, op. cit., p. 26.
13. Single Mothers by Choice, brochure, New York.
14. Robinson, op. cit., p. 3.
15. Kirkendall and Whitehurst, op. cit., p. 9.
16. Carson Strong, "The Single Woman and Artificial Insemination by Donor," *The Journal of Reproductive Medicine*, Vol. 29, No. 5, May 1984. p. 295.

17. James Barron, "View on Surrogacy after Baby M Ruling," *New York Times*, April 2, 1987.
18. "American Survey," *Economist*, May 31, 1986.
19. Leonard Groopman, "Letter to the Editor", *New York Times*, April 12, 1987.
20. Rhonda Billig, presentation to American Civil Liberties Union, Washington D.C., June 24, 1987.
21. Ibid.
22. Quoted in Cyril C. Means Jr., "Surrogacy versus the Thirteenth Amendment," presentation at American Bay Association Annual Meeting, August 1987, p. 17.
23. Ibid., p. 19.
24. Ibid., p. 18.
25. Ibid., p. 18.
26. AP: "Surrogate has baby conceived in laboratory," *New York Times* April 17, 1986.
27. Stacy DeBroff, National Staff Surrogate Paper for ACLU, June 24, 1987.
28. John Ray, "Consumer Protection and Regulation of Surrogate Parenting Centers Act of 1987, Bill 7-176," March 24, 1987.
29. *Economist*, July 14, 1984.
30. Charles Krauthammer, "The Ethics of Human Manufacturing," *The New Republic*, May 4, 1987.
31. Jeremy Rifkin, *Algeny: A New Word—A New World*, New York, Penguin Books, 1984. p. 50.
32. Ibid., p. 52.
33. Linda Salzer, *Infertility, How Couples can Cope*, G.K. Hall & Co., Mass, 1986, p. 32–33.
34. Corea, op. cit., pp. 123–124.
35. Germaine Greer, *Sex and Destiny: Politics of Human Fertility*, Harper and Row, New York, 1984, p. 6.
36. Quoted in Peter Singer and Deane Wells, *Making Babies*, New York, Charles Scribner's Sons, 1985, p. 125.
37. Quoted in Corea, Russell Scott, *The Body as Property*, New York, Viking Press, 1981, p. 41.
38. Quoted in Singer and Wells, p. 121.
39. Ibid., p. 125.
40. Clifford Grobstein, *From Chance to Purpose: An appraisal of External Human Fertilization*. Reading, Massachusetts, Addison-Wesley Publishing Company, 1981, p. XII.
41. John Edsall, "Biology and Human Values" in Walter J. Org., ed., *Knowledge and the Future of Man*, New York, Holt Reinchart & Winston, 1968, p. 159.
42. Rifkin, op. cit., p. 53.

43. Daniel J. Kevles: *In the Name of Eugenics*, University of California Press, Berkeley, 1985, p. 289.
44. Ibid., p. 286.
45. Boston Women's Health Book Collective, *The New Our Bodies Ourselves*, New York, Simon and Shuster, 1984.
46. Kevles, op. cit., p. 291.
47. Ellen Perley Frank "Greater Expectations," *Washington Post Magazine*, June 2, 1985.
48. Food and Drug Administration, "FDA Talk Paper", Jan. 21, 1987.
49. Kelves, op. cit., pp. 292–293.
50. Ibid., p. 293.
51. Ibid., p. 288.
52. Ruth Hubbard and Judy Norsigian, "Genetic Screening, Theology and Abortion and Reproduction Choice," Forum on Reproductive Laws for the 1990s, Rutgers University, May, 1987.
53. Richard Cohen, "A Child of One's Own" *Washington Post Magazine*, February 15, 1987.
54. Martha Weinman Lear, *The Child Worshipers*, New York, Crown Publishers, Inc., 1963, p. 132.
55. Philippe Ariès, *Centuries of childhood: A Social History of Family Life*, New York, Vintage Books, 1962, p. 38.
56. Ibid., page 39.
57. Melvin Konner. A Tangled Wing: Biological Constraints on the Human Spirit, New York, Holt, Rienhard & Winston, 1982, pp. 291–2.

EPILOGUE

1. Lester Kirkendall and Robert Whitehurst, eds., *The New Sexual Revolution*, New York, Donald W. Brown, Inc., New York, Inc., 1971, p. 198.

Index